SEARCHING FOR THE FAMILY DOCTOR

SEARCHING FOR THE FAMILY DOCTOR

Primary Care on the Brink

TIMOTHY J. HOFF

JOHNS HOPKINS UNIVERSITY PRESS | *Baltimore*

© 2022 Timothy J. Hoff
All rights reserved. Published 2022
Printed in the United States of America on acid-free paper
9 8 7 6 5 4 3 2 1

Johns Hopkins University Press
2715 North Charles Street
Baltimore, Maryland 21218-4363
www.press.jhu.edu

Library of Congress Cataloging-in-Publication Data

Names: Hoff, Timothy, 1965– author.
Title: Searching for the family doctor : primary care on the brink /
    Timothy J. Hoff.
Description: Baltimore : Johns Hopkins University Press, 2022. | Includes
    bibliographical references and index.
Identifiers: LCCN 2021017978 | ISBN 9781421443003 (hardcover) |
    ISBN 9781421443010 (ebook)
Subjects: LCSH: Primary care (Medicine)—United States. | Family
    medicine—United States.
Classification: LCC RA427.9 .H642 2022 | DDC 362.10973—dc23
LC record available at https://lccn.loc.gov/2021017978
A catalog record for this book is available from the British Library.

*Special discounts are available for bulk purchases of this book. For more
information, please contact Special Sales at specialsales@jh.edu.*

To my wife Sharon, and son Kieran, who are
everything to me

I am a Family Physician,
one of many across this country.

This is what I believe:
You, the patient, are my first professional responsibility whether man or woman
or child, ill or well, seeking care, healing, or knowledge.

You and your family deserve high-quality, affordable health care including
treatment, prevention, and health promotion.

I support access to health care for all.

The specialty of family practice trains me to care for the whole person physically
and emotionally, throughout life, working with your medical history and family
dynamics, coordinating your care with other physicians when necessary.

This is my promise to you.

The Family Physician's Creed

CONTENTS

The Family Doctor's Role in the Primary Care War

There is a fight going on for the soul of not only American health care but health care everywhere. Primary care is at the center of this struggle, the essence of which is the unresolved tension between two different goals. One goal is a fair, empathic, and highly relational care delivery system, built around primary care and trusting relationships between doctors and patients. Another goal is a more efficient, convenient, and highly transactional care delivery system, impersonal and built on algorithms, health care corporations, and technology. The former needs family doctors to succeed. The latter probably does not, relying instead on business thinking, scale, cheap labor, and technology.

Make no mistake, this is an escalating war with combatants joining both sides. The COVID-19 pandemic has accelerated it by providing further rationales for minimizing the imperfect equation of using humans in health care delivery and embracing the transition to technological solutions instead. This will be a war that is fought in health care over the next several decades, and there will be lots of casualties. One combatant fighting on the side of relational primary care and the role of doctors, particularly general doctors, is the specialty of family medicine. Born out of the chaos and opportunity of 1960s America, this specialty has tried to position itself at the center of primary care medicine in the United States. For over fifty years, it has been selling us the idea that a comprehensive physician who can manage care and who sees all patients as unique, whole individuals has immense value. This specialty has grown since the late 1960s, has had success, has been bogged down, has languished at times and briefly flourished again, and now exists in a precarious state. It has experienced an ongoing identity crisis related to what it wants to be and can be in our health care system. But it remains vulnerable to assaults from health care corporations and technology companies seeking health care as the next profit-making frontier.

There are approximately 223,000 primary care physicians in the United States, which is almost one-third of all physicians. Almost 90,000 of these primary care physicians are family doctors (Peterson et al. 2018). It sounds like a lot, but it is nowhere near enough to bring the vision of the generalist doctor and holistic care to everyone in America. These foot soldiers of the primary care army are turned out annually into a medical specialty that has tried in the past to pitch itself as "counter-culture," providing pushback against the overly procedural, highly specialized, and fragmented care delivery system which has been ascendant since the 1960s.

It does not seem like a fair fight in many ways for 90,000 family doctors scattered across the United States to take on even larger numbers of procedural specialists, the Amazons and Apples, and big health care organizations that tower like moated castle kingdoms over our country's landscape. It is an army that cannot seem to grow any larger, whose core identity is suspect, whose ranks are balkanized, and whose resources and control on the ground weaken with each passing day. Especially over the past couple of decades, when the health care system in America continued to underpay for and underinvest in primary care, encouraged system fragmentation that makes the family doctor's job harder, and became enamored with technology and retail thinking.

Why should we be interested in this war and who wins? Why should we care about the future of family doctors as a viable army to win the war for the side of physician-centric, primary care medicine? On a big-picture level, health care is another example in modern society of a service industry overrun by "innovators" thinking they can provide better care for patients than doctors. Doctors are under threat and increasingly marginalized through the "Amazoning" of health care, where the large corporation controls everything upstream and downstream in the production process. Family doctors are first in the crosshairs of that powerful idea because family doctors stand in the way of big organizations taking over health care. As these doctors go, so may go other types of doctors—along with the notion of a health care delivery system with the physician-patient relationship and physician expertise at its core. The ideal of a comprehensive or generalist doctor who can manage our care and needs holistically could vanish.

These types of doctors, and the primary care medicine they practice, are eminently important for all of us to lead longer, happier, and healthier lives. The research shows that, as does common sense. The kind of medicine family doctors dispense is focused on preventing disease, keeping individuals healthy, improving the health of communities, and taking care of health problems before they spiral into bigger problems. The best family doctor–patient relationships have high degrees of interpersonal trust, empathy, mutual respect, and loyalty. These features have been shown over time to be vital to improving people's health. It is not just the kind of medicine that counts. It is the human-to-human bonds that family doctors form with their patients which positively impact patient care. It is the notion of health care as a humane enterprise, typified not by decisions around what is most efficient and least costly but rather around what is most caring and conducive to patient needs. This is why the war is so important.

Unfortunately, the specialty of family medicine is not prepared for this war, and the army it currently trains and supports in the field is not prepared to take on the fight. It is an army weakened by decades of compromises, rigid ideology, too much of a copycat mentality, an inability to adapt to the changing terrain and take advantage of it when afforded the opportunity, and poorer preparation for the various battles being fought daily in health settings across America. This book explores that reality and presents a case for why it might be so, focusing on the army itself and the strategic decision making of its early leadership. It also focuses on the foot soldiers expected to wage this fight, and what they have had to do to make their careers sustainable.

This book does not analyze the war itself. My 2017 book *Next in Line* does some of that. Instead, it uses historical and current-day perspectives to analyze how the specialty of family medicine has evolved to where it is today. This evolution matters if we want to understand why primary care in the United States has languished over time, why it remains subservient to other types of medicine, and whether it can reassert itself as the most important and well-funded aspect of our health care system. Through the voices of current family doctors young and old, and the voices of those family doctors long gone, we hear the individual stories that inform the story of primary care—how the specialty has evolved and what that means for its current members, its patients, and its survival.

I do not offer a simple or fully optimistic picture of how family medicine can be saved, or how its ranks can be made stronger. Rather, I provide a blunt yet informed take on a specialty that started and grew in a certain way. Not in an inevitable way mind you, but rather a deliberate, strategic way guided by real people exerting their power and influence to make things happen. This analysis, while acknowledging that the American health care system—in all its dysfunctional glory—has been inhospitable to the growth and survival of family medicine, turns the spotlight on the specialty itself: its early history, its early leaders and strategies, and the experiences and choices of its own rank and file. It is a critical, much-needed review that seeks to explain how family medicine got into a mess largely of its own accord—and what it may take to save it. A vibrant family medicine specialty makes the prospect of a high-quality health system with greater equality that much more possible.

Why is a book with this type of perspective needed? Because the story warrants it. By focusing on how family medicine and family doctors have put themselves in an unenviable position with regard to being able to make our health care system better, I am doing what most other writers and researchers interested in health care choose not to do. One need only look up some titles on Amazon to see book after book with pretty much the same theme espoused: health care has been taken over by the profiteers who plan on ruining it. These include insurance companies, tech companies, hospitals, entrepreneurs, and monopolistic care delivery systems like those that flourish in my backyard of Boston, Massachusetts. These other works, however, while often well researched and powerful in their prose, rarely assess the physician's part in the story. This makes our understanding of any story in health care incomplete. In addition, it is always interesting to examine how any entity, especially one filled from top to bottom with very smart people, does things that come back to haunt it. Studying elite professionals like doctors is an exercise in gaining appreciation for how all occupational groups pursue self-interest, and how that self-interest can benefit societal interests but also wreak havoc on the occupation's members and their everyday existence.

This book relies on historical and ethnographic data. It is neither a complete history of the family medicine specialty, nor is it only a qualitative study of a group of family doctors. I think the strength of the book's direction and analysis lie in the fact that the historical data mixes with the interview data. This mixing creates a story that is at once "in real time" and grounded in the early evolution and decision making of the specialty and its key leaders, giving it context and perspective. If you want to know where you are and where you are going, know where you have been. For example, when you are reading about a current group of family doctors who are trying to pursue sustainable careers and make job choices that are not aligned with the comprehensive family doctor ideal, you are also hearing about how certain strategic choices the specialty made back in the late 1960s and early 1970s might have influenced the behavior of those family doctors.

Any book like this, using data like this, tries to create a compelling argument for why something is the way it is. Of course, that argument is more or less convincing depending on how the author has tried to interpret the data and the manner in which they have constructed the architecture of the argument. Personally, having done many research studies in my career, I really like the data upon which the arguments in this book are based. They tend to triangulate the main points in a way that is believable and richly detailed. For example, when you read about the issues around identity, imitation, and the definitions drawn from the historical data, and then you subsequently read about the struggles that individuals go through to construct their identities and roles as family doctors on an everyday basis, it does not seem all that surprising that the two are linked. Of course, one of the main jobs of the researcher is to obtain and analyze the data to make that linkage for the reader, offering it up for their consideration. The historical and ethnographic data for this book were extensive and rich enough to make that job difficult but eminently doable.

Before moving onto this story, special thanks are in order. First, and most important, are the thanks due to my wife, Sharon, and our 14-year-old son, Kieran. A good chunk of this book was researched and written during the COVID-19 pandemic, particularly the several months' long shutdown that required all of us to essentially remain in our homes full-time. Everyone knows, especially those with young children, what a stressful time this was, and I did not always have the energy and free time to sit down and finish a major research project and book manuscript. There were days I was too tired, too aggravated, too down, or too busy (or all of the above) to summon up meaningful energy on this project. Other times it did not seem that important. But I was able to gather myself over time, and it was largely because of their support.

My son took on his responsibilities for online schooling with a professionalism and maturity I have not seen in many adults I know. He kept himself busy enough of the time to allow me to go upstairs to my office and write. He is quite the young man. My wife, Sharon, who has been my companion for over thirty-five years, was also working from home, and she did what she always does, which is everything. Taking care of us, working a difficult job, helping my son get through that forgettable period of school, and keeping our house in order. That allowed me to dither more on something (this book) that frankly pales in importance to what all of us have gone through during 2020. I do not write any books without her support.

Other thanks are also due. Thanks to the Center for History in Family Medicine (CHFM), and its parent the American Academy of Family Physicians Foundation, for giving me access to the CHFM archives—what a special repository of important historical information on the US medical profession, family medicine, and the primary care system. I am not a historian, but visiting the CHFM and having days to look through the stacks for many different things has made me feel like I might want to become one. The center's leadership, including Crystal Bauer and Don

Ivey, was both helpful and supportive, helping me figure out what I should be looking at and where I could find it.

There were fifty-five different family doctors I interviewed for this book, some more than once, who also deserve many thanks. I have interviewed hundreds of physicians in my research career, but there is no group more amiable and interesting to talk with than family doctors. They are some of the nicest and best human beings I have had the opportunity to meet. They gave time out of their busy workdays to be interviewed, and this book would not have happened without them. I tell any researchers who will listen that if you want to understand health care, talk to doctors. Doctors know things. They are at the center of it all. Many of them also think about their work lives and what they do quite deeply. I knew from the outset that a story about family medicine had to include the perspectives and experiences of its doctors. They had to help tell the story.

Several of those with whom I spoke have also been included in my other research studies looking at different questions. Others were doctors with whom I spoke for the first time. Several allowed me to interview them more than once. Almost all let me ask questions that gravitated toward the personal, such as why they became doctors and family doctors, how they thought about and made career and job choices, what they liked and did not like about being a family doctor, aspects of their home lives, and how they performed their everyday work roles. The New York State Academy of Family Physicians, and their leadership, was instrumental in helping me gain access to the physicians I interviewed. They are a great organization with great people. I cannot thank them enough for their help and patience. Thanks also to Johns Hopkins University Press and my editor, Robin Coleman, who saw value in this story and was very helpful in providing feedback that made it a readable one.

SEARCHING FOR THE FAMILY DOCTOR

ONE

Searching for the Family Doctor

Fayette has a new doctor. He is Dr. R.O. Rutland, Jr. who established practice at the McNease-clinic Monday. A Native of Eufaula, Dr. Rutland graduated from high school there and finished in pre-medicine at the University of Alabama. He attended the medical school at Tulane University and received his internship at Jefferson-Hillman hospital in Birmingham. After serving as a doctor in the U.S. Navy two years, Dr. Rutland spent two years in general practice residency, one of which was in California and one in Colorado. "I plan to stay in small town practice the rest of my life," the young doctor said. Fayette is his first small town private practice and he says he thinks he will like it here.

Fayette, Alabama, local paper, August 1954 (Rutland Papers, Center for the History of Family Medicine [CHFM])

Like many small town boys, I idolized my family doctor. My admiration went beyond the fact that in medical matters he was to me omnipotent. It reflected a close personal feeling which developed through the years he treated my family and me and lived a leader's role in our community. My folks always said that this great adulation started when, treating me during a bad spell of diphtheria when I was four, he gave me a silver dollar. There allegedly followed a promise that "When I grow up," every effort would be made to follow in those footsteps and maybe spread a few silver dollars around. It made a good story.

> Richard Rutland, 1962, "The Family Doctor's 'Return' " (Rutland Papers, CHFM)

"A fine physician, conscientious and capable, with a deep sense of humility and responsibility to his patients and the community"—those were the words used by the president of the Alabama Academy of Family Physicians to describe Richard O. Rutland, M.D., of Fayette, Ala., chosen by Good Housekeeping and the American Academy of Family Physicians as the 1981 Family Doctor of the Year. This is the fifth year that Good Housekeeping and the academy have joined to honor those physicians who are dedicated to serving their communities by maintaining the highest standards in medical care.

> *Good Housekeeping* magazine, 1981 (Rutland Papers, CHFM)

Dear Dr. Rutland,
Congratulations on your retirement. You really deserve some time off. One of my first and best memories of you is August 23, 1968 when you delivered my son because Dr. Breitling was out of town. Another memory I am very grateful for is all the years you were my dear mother's doctor. She was so proud of you when you won the Good Housekeeping Award. She cut out the article and showed it to everyone who came to see her. You always made her feel better and lifted her spirits even in the last days when nothing medically would help her.

> Karen L.
> Patient letter to Dr. Rutland upon his retirement, 1997 (Rutland Papers, CHFM)

As a small-town physician, you deal with people whose names you know. You live with your patients, go to church with them, share an interest in your children's schools and the civic and social life of your community. I have looked after people for 20 to 25 years, and in many cases their children and even their grandchildren. And there is a personal warmth between the small-town doctor and the patients he treats that comes from a sense of continuing care.

Richard Rutland, 1981, *Good Housekeeping* magazine (Rutland Papers, CHFM)

IF DR. RICHARD RUTLAND, *Good Housekeeping* magazine's 1981 Family Doctor of the Year, was starting out today, there is a good chance he would not choose to become a family doctor at all but a higher-paid surgeon or other type of specialist. If he did choose family medicine, there is a strong possibility that instead of being a small-town, self-employed family doctor with a loyal, long-standing group of patients, he would work as a nine-to-five salaried employee for a hospital system or spread-out network of cookie-cutter primary care practices, with patients churning in and out of his practice on a frequent basis as their insurance and employers changed. He might be working in an urgent care center, maybe doing part-time work in a couple of different clinical jobs at once to get more time off or help pay down his student loan debt quicker. Or he could be a hospitalist, one of those doctors who take care of patients while they are in the hospital.

He might seek out the presumed haven of an academic family medicine position, partially sheltered from the harsher realities of modern family practice, where he would be underpaid but maintain some perceived variety in his work. He might not be doing full-time clinical work at all, but instead would be employed in an administrative position managing other physicians, as a medical director, or doing quality-improvement work. There is a good possibility that over the course of his career, he would find himself taking several different jobs along the way, relocating several times in the process, and leaving his existing patients more than once over a twenty- or thirty-year period of practice.

The Richard Rutland of today would need to make his career choices carefully. He would quickly feel trapped in a health care system inhospitable to primary care work and family medicine careers. He would see burned-out mentors and dissatisfied colleagues working too hard for too little. That would scare him at the outset of his own career. He would see less payment for his services than he would like. He would see patients who increasingly want convenience and speed in getting their primary care services, who have fewer experiences with a regular family doctor, and who are told by the health care marketplace that the very idea of having the same primary care doctor over time is outdated and unnecessary.

He would also probably wonder a lot more about what it was he was supposed to do each day as a family doctor. Given all the job and employment-setting choices available to him, watching his family medicine colleagues take different kinds of jobs, and seeing his specialty advocating for family doctors to work not only as full-scope generalists in ambulatory care settings but also as hospitalists and emergency room doctors that provide only a piece of the generalist role, he might get confused about his role very quickly.

In this sense, the Richard Rutland of today would be part of a specialty experiencing a profound identity crisis—struggling for relevance, perhaps survival, amid ongoing attacks from other specialties bent on carving up the family doctor job description. He would be working amid a plague-like spread of "pop-up" primary care alternatives for patients, such as urgent care centers; a growing belief that algorithmic care through technological innovations like smartphone apps can deliver good, timely primary care without doctors; and a greater use of nurse practitioners and physician assistants in every primary care setting (Hoff 2017; Landi 2019).

The Richard Rutland of yesteryear considered himself a "family doctor." He never wavered from making the town of Fayette, Alabama, his home and workplace for the duration of his long career as a physician. Fayette, a poorer rural town of a few thousand people sitting in the central western part of Alabama, has rarely seen more than 5,000 people living in it. Almost 20 percent of its citizenry live below the poverty line today, and its median household income is less than $30,000 per year. Fayette boasts the largest glove manufacturing plant in America these days, and it is home to Ox Bodies, a leader in the construction and sale of dump truck bodies (City of Fayette 2019). Geographically, it sits less than an hour north of Tuscaloosa, home of the famous University of Alabama

Crimson Tide football team, placing it at the epicenter of the grand tradition of college football in the United States. The town got its first paved road in 1926 and its first hospital in 1938 (City of Fayette 2019). What it has never had a lot of are doctors. When Richard Rutland came to town in 1954, he was a needed asset for the people of Fayette, who welcomed him. They understood his value to them and the community.

As a Tulane University medical school graduate and recent general practice resident, Rutland came to Fayette with his wife, Nancy, and two small children to learn surgery under a fellow colleague. He did not plan to stay there. Yet, like many turns that life takes, he stayed longer. He was a small-town boy himself, growing up in another part of rural Alabama in a town called Eufaula. There was a lot to like about staying in Fayette given his background. It felt right. Unburdened by the financial debt of going to medical school, having a growing family, and able to become a central figure in the health care of the Fayette community right away, Fayette could give a family doctor like Rutland autonomy, respect, and the potential for a rewarding career.

Like the general practitioner of old, his scope of medical practice was large and varied. He got to know and treat entire families. He did everything: delivered babies, helped people die, took care of young children, treated chronic diseases, dispensed prevention and lifestyle advice, comforted the afflicted, treated depression, performed minor surgeries and procedures, cared for patients in the hospital and intensive care unit, treated entire families, developed and read X-rays, coordinated and managed his patients' care with other specialists when needed, and conducted detailed physical exams and patient histories that allowed him to arrive at appropriate diagnoses and treatment plans. He listened to patients and spent time with them. He tried to heal, educate, advise, and support them all at once.

April 7, 1997

Dear Dr. Rutland:
Thank you for the care you have given both Leslie and me during the past several years. When we moved back to Fayette after living in Mobile for many, many years, you helped to make this big transition an easier

one for us. Leslie was already a sick man, but you looked after him until his death in December 1994.

As for myself, you helped guide me through this most difficult time in my life. Not only did I have to learn to live without my life's mate, but at 82 years of age, I had to learn to live alone. You urged me (very strongly I might add) to give the "Life Line" a try, and I did. I have learned to become self-sufficient with the loving care of family, friends, and a good doctor like you.

Not only have you treated me when I was physically ill, but best of all you have been my friend and given me emotional support at some of the lowest times of my life. I will miss your loving care, but you need time to enjoy your life with your family without the cares and demands of others. I wish you and your lovely wife well during this new experience of life.

Effie B.

Patient letter to Dr. Rutland upon his retirement, 1997 (Rutland Papers, CHFM)

June 26, 1997

Dear Dr. Rutland,

I don't really know how many years I have been your patient but quite a few. I have always thought you were the "greatest." Not only have you been a great doctor but you have been my friend, my confidant, and I appreciate that so much. You always took time to listen to my "woes" and gave me good advice. I can't say I always followed the advice but it was good. I believe you to be "one of a kind." I will miss you greatly and so will all your patients.

Sincerely, Fay

Patient letter to Dr. Rutland upon his retirement, 1997 (Rutland Papers, CHFM)

He was also there for his patients, day in and day out, as they grew old with him:

Dr. Rutland,

Through the years that you've been my doctor, you've also been my best friend. You've given me advice so many times when it was needed just as you gave me medicine for whatever was wrong with me. All the years Ed was sick I always knew I could depend on you to help me in so many ways. When it seemed sometimes I would go no farther you always had the right words to say to lift me up. I'll miss you so much, just enjoy your retirement, you have earned every minute of it.

Martha D.

Patient letter to Dr. Rutland upon his retirement, 1997 (Rutland Papers, CHFM)

To a dear friend,

On July 27, 1973, I had an accident. You were at the emergency room at the Fayette County Hospital and you and God saved my life. I would like to thank you for always being there for me. You have been my friend and my doctor ever since. I will miss you dearly when you retire.

Billy W.

Patient letter to Dr. Rutland upon his retirement, 1997 (Rutland Papers, CHFM)

Dear Dr. Rutland,

I thank you for the thorough way you cared for me when I got sick, when I had seizures and fainting spells. I think you are the best doctor in the whole world and I know you and Nancy will enjoy doing things like traveling, taking it easy, and just enjoying yourselves. You are such a good friend, Dr. Rutland, and you are always easy to talk to. Thank you for the insurance you got me at Lanier Clothes, for getting me to the doctors to let me have check-ups. You did not give up on getting me the plant insurance and that's what I will remember most about it! I wish you and Nancy best wishes on your retirement! I love you!

Jack

Patient letter to Dr. Rutland upon his retirement, 1997 (Rutland Papers, CHFM)

To be this kind of doctor he sacrificed important things in his own life, as did his family. This was a necessary part of being the full-scope generalist. Work was on his mind or at his fingertips most of the time. He left his family in the middle of the night to go to patients' houses.

He ducked out of movies and restaurants to get to the hospital and check on someone in the intensive care unit or to deliver a baby. He missed school events and family parties. He didn't keep a watch on his work. Medicine was a true round-the-clock calling, not a nine-to-five job, at least to Richard Rutland. This was part of the bargain he made in becoming a family doctor.

> Getting up at 5 a.m. is "old hat" for Dr. Richard O. Rutland Jr. As a family doctor in Fayette, he has been doing it for years, seeing patients, holding staff meetings, performing a number of professional and civic duties, deliver[ing] babies—some 1,800 of them at last count—and even making house calls. . . . One of his few regrets in the past 25 years, says the physician, is that his practice and other duties have kept him away from his family too much. "Credit for raising the children has to go mainly to their mother," he readily adds. "That has been my most difficult problem—how to devote enough time to my practice, my family, myself and my community."
>
> *Birmingham News*, August 27, 1981 (Rutland Papers, CHFM)

There was something Richard Rutland and those like him gained in making this bargain though—something immeasurably valuable. That was the happiness and personal satisfaction associated with being a real part of people's everyday lives, there with them during both good times and bad. The Richard Rutland of today would have much less opportunity, for many reasons, to derive this joy and satisfaction from his patients. Today, he would see most of his patients only when something was wrong. These encounters, time limited and devoid of pleasantries, would leave little room for the sort of small talk that bonds doctors and patients together. He would have only a few minutes with each of them. There would be fewer opportunities and little incentive to celebrate a patient's newborn child, pay raise, or son's or daughter's latest report card. There would be less of a reason to share in their good times, no matter how small, because he was no longer one of them, a trusted friend as well as a doctor. Without this genuine aspect of his everyday work, one that a part of him craved as the biggest reward of being a doctor, the difficult bargain he made with his profession would seem less worth it, begging the question of whether he would indeed make such a bargain at all.

When Family Doctors Were Called General Practitioners

There were many other doctors fifty years ago who made such a bargain. Called *general practitioners* (GPs), they were the backbone of health care delivery, particularly in the small towns and rural areas of America. Glorified during an earlier time as the "horse and buggy doctor," who in many rural towns were the only ones to turn to when sick, they were the healers who would visit people in their homes at all hours and in all weather, dispensing medicine, kindness, and compassion (Hertzler and Stone 1938). Many did not have the most advanced clinical training. Nor was there generally a lot of advanced clinical training to be had. Most GPs instead excelled in the science of understanding people. A big part of their job was comforting patients, listening to them, offering them advice, and helping them and their families through the most difficult times of their lives. What they lacked in clinical acumen was often made up for through years of on-the-job training in the art of the human condition, and high doses of emotional intelligence.

The iconic image of the GP in America hung around for a long time, through almost all of the twentieth century, despite the explosion in medical science and the concomitant turn toward high-cost, procedure-happy doctors and super specialists who dealt more with specific body parts than whole persons. In 1970, the television show *Marcus Welby, M.D.* won the Emmy Award for best TV drama and Robert Young, in the role of the title character, won the Emmy for best dramatic performance. It was one of the highest-rated television shows of the early 1970s. Welby was a GP molded in the spirit of the generalist doctor that never turned away a patient, one who devoted all of his time to his craft, used little technology, and diagnosed and treated a full range of maladies—physical and mental.

At a time when medical specialization was taking over American medicine and the glitz of new, high-priced technologies like the CT scan began infiltrating health care delivery, millions of American TV viewers tuned in each week to watch Welby and his younger sidekick, Dr. Kiley, ply their trades in a simpler, more humane manner. They listened, spent time with patients, took an interest in their lives, and were compassionate yet honest.

Like Richard Rutland, television doctor Marcus Welby and his protégé, played by James Brolin, believed that relational excellence mattered a great deal in being an effective family doctor. To them, knowing people helped to diagnose and treat physical illness. They saw their jobs also as ensuring patients' spiritual and emotional well-being, helping them become happier and get through their days easier, and preventing things like illness from occurring in the first place if possible. They treated patients holistically, as living beings with prior histories and current life contexts. They gave advice. They listened. They tried to help. The work of a good GP, a true family doctor in the Welby general practitioner mold, was as much motivational for patients as it was anything else.

General practitioners relied on their personality and experience knowing a given patient to extract important information that could help them understand who and what was presenting before them. For example, there was no electronic health record to serve as a repository for the patient's information, or to use for managing their care. There were no standardized quality metrics and few evidence-based care guidelines to follow. No computer algorithms were spitting out preferred treatment pathways and neutering the family doctor's ability to use their experience and understanding of a single patient to give the best care. A limited number of laboratory tests, targeted medications, and expensive diagnostic devices were available. Patients controlled their health care information because most of it resided inside of their own heads. GPs were responsible for extracting it in full if they wanted to provide good care. No smartphone app or Apple Watch was going to get it for them.

Beyond the clinical value it offered, GPs believed knowing their patients intimately was an important part of their identities as family doctors. It was who they were as professionals. It was both an obligation and necessity of delivering holistic medicine—a clinician who viewed health and disease through the lens of the entire person and their everyday life. This approach sees patients as unique rather than alike, individuals whose family, community, and environmental contexts affect their health and ability to take proper care of themselves. To care holistically for a patient and be an effective generalist was to understand something about these contexts for every patient. Therefore, seeing the same patients, living in the same community, and caring for entire families for a long period of time, as well as taking an active personal interest in improving the surrounding environment, was a natural part of being a good GP.

These doctors saw their patients at church or at the local supermarket or restaurant. Their kids went to the same schools and they participated in school councils and town book clubs together. They treated them holistically because they saw them as fully formed human beings with lives of their own and children, spouses, and everyday experiences that were unique to them. This intimacy gave them a personal and professional reason for knowing them—for not wanting to see them any more unhappy or unhealthy than they wanted to see themselves or their own family. In this way, being a general practitioner and a family doctor was ideally a societal endeavor that placed these professionals at the nexus of a larger citizenry in the surrounding environs. It made many of these physicians, ones like Richard Rutland, more willing to enact their roles in a way that brought them closer to their patients' lives and required significant expertise in human skills such as providing empathy and compassion, being a good listener, and showing respect and admiration.

> What of this close doctor-patient relationship, is it real? Not always but usually. How can I as a family doctor be impersonal about a patient whose grandpa and cousins are acquaintances if not friends of mine; whose work, whose likes and dislikes, strengths and weaknesses are part of my background knowledge of him? The proximity of our lives is close in many respects. Certainly, I have a personal interest which often develops into a warm relationship.
>
> Richard Rutland, 1962, "The Family Doctor's 'Return'" (Rutland Papers, CHFM)

April 7, 1997

Dear Dr. Rutland:

Let me say "thank you" for all you have done for my family and to tell you what a pleasure it has been just being associated with you. Thank God for you being there during our sick days, our sad days, during our great health days and our happiest days (the grandchildren). Thank you for letting me and Rocky be just a small part of your career. Not only at the clinic but also at the Fayette County Hospital.

Speaking for my family, my parents, Gene and myself, Rocky and David our children, Lane and Adam our grandchildren and other members of my family[,] we shall forever be so grateful for your being there for us. . . . You became the doctor and a great individual for whom we had so much respect, trust, appreciation and admiration. . . . You have helped to make our lives more important to us as individuals. Thank you for being there to comfort us, to give us medical attention, just to talk. It seemed our concerns were also your concerns. Thank you for your professionalism, outstanding attitude and your dedication to not only our family but to all your patients.

My family and I know everyone in town feel that you have been such a great asset to the community and the medical field. All your accomplishments will be rewarded hopefully by being able to spend time with your children, grandchildren, and all the other things you choose to do.

Our family will never forget you. What will we do now?

Eugene and Florence F.

P.S. Continue with much happiness but be sure to stay active and watch the calories.

Patient letter to Dr. Rutland upon his retirement, 1997 (Rutland Papers, CHFM)

To watch reruns of *Marcus Welby* is to be amazed by how much he and his partner were involved in their patients' lives, and how much patients often wanted them to be involved, or at least ultimately benefitted from that involvement. In one second-season episode entitled "A Very Special Sailfish," one of Welby's teenage female patients contracts a sexually transmitted disease and demurs from telling her parents. She also holds back from Welby information about the partner from whom she contracted the disease. This is a patient and family it seems Welby has known forever. The parents are having a difficult time understanding their daughter's circumstances, and she is reticent to open up to them. Welby goes out of his way to visit the hospital where she ends up, not only caring for her but also providing emotional support and friendly advice. He gets her to talk honestly with him and tries to talk her through her best options. He also visits her parents several times at their home to listen to their anxieties about raising their daughter, comfort them, and even offer a bit of marriage counseling in the process.

Hollywood fantasy at its finest? Perhaps. After all, looking through the lens of 2020 America, when it takes months in many locales to get a new patient appointment with a primary care doctor; where it is nearly impossible to see your regular family physician, if you are lucky enough to have one, without waiting days or weeks; where most primary care offices shutter completely at 5 p.m. until the next day and do not take any calls on the weekend; and where many primary care doctors leave one practice after another on a frequent basis, severing themselves from their patients, it is difficult to imagine that there were many doctors who willingly took on these types of roles with their patients (Hoff 2010; Merritt Hawkins 2017).

Richard Rutland did, and others did too. It was not only the product of a fictional television show.

> Dear Dr. Rutland,
> I would just like to thank you for the wonderful care you gave my husband Leonard. I know he was not the most cooperative patient, but you seemed to understand. Thanks for talking to me so I could understand. And thanks most of all for just being where I needed you.
> Sincerely, Sarah E.
> Patient letter to Dr. Rutland upon his retirement, 1997 (Rutland Papers, CHFM)

Richard Rutland did things in Fayette he would have never done had he only stayed a few years and then moved. If he had moved from one employer to another frequently. If he had been working as a salaried employee of some larger corporate health care system. Or if he had simply decided he wanted to work nine-to-five each day and spend his nights and weekends doing other things. He did things for the community as a family doctor because he was a permanent part of the community, and the community mattered to him.

> The Eufaula native [Dr. Rutland] has been a driving force behind the family doctor concept from the time he, his wife Nancy and their children chose Fayette as their place in 1954. And he was instrumental in organizing and starting the state's present program of educating and training physicians for family practice, with particular emphasis on serving in rural areas. . . . Rutland, his fellow doctors and Fayette built McNease-Hodo Medical Clinic, generally recognized as one of the most modern rural clinics in the state. It was built with the hope of attracting more physicians. The community is particularly in need of another surgeon, says Rutland. Rutland also was instrumental in establishing a smaller clinic in [the] 800-population Community of Berry, 18 miles away in east Fayette County. For years he drove to Berry on his "day off" to see patients after the community lost its only doctor in the early 1970s. "The new clinic in Fayette is something he had dreamed of, I suppose, since he came here," said Bob Sanders, a Fayette insurance executive and close friend. "If Doc had died the day the clinic was dedicated, he'd have died happy."
> *Birmingham News*, August 27, 1981 (Rutland Papers, CHFM)

As he mastered his art in rural family practice, Dr. Rutland's influence expanded through the community and the medical profession. Because of their confidence in him, his peers propelled him to leadership in the state's family physicians' organization. In 1961, he was elected president of the Alabama Chapter of the American Academy of Family Physicians. While serving in this capacity, he became concerned about the growing trend among newly educated physicians to sub-specialize, instead of pursuing general practice. His childhood role model and his experience caring for Fayette confirmed for him that physicians who were broadly trained to care for the large majority of health care concerns experienced by most patients was the principal medical education need in the state. He expressed this view and looked for the opportunity to lead Alabama's medical education program in this direction.

When fourth year medical student Lee Taylor in Birmingham started the push for a clinical rotation in an outlying area, Dr. Rutland was quick to respond. In 1966, he worked with the University of Alabama School of Medicine, located in Birmingham, to have Fayette approved as a preceptor site for fourth-year medical students. In the fifteen years that followed, almost fifty students and family practice residents took clinical rotations in Fayette, learning from accomplished local physicians in their offices, the hospital, and community settings. The people of Fayette were proud partners in the effort to produce physicians who understood the lives of rural Alabamians and were prepared to serve them.

When need for family doctors for rural areas became an issue in Alabama in the late 1960s, Dr. Rutland was an acknowledged leader in this field. Soon he was enlisted by the University of Alabama in the effort to establish a new medical education program for that purpose. In 1969, UA President David Matthews involved him and Dr. John Burnum, a Tuscaloosa Internist, in planning and recruiting a dean to establish the College of Community Health Sciences (CCHS) and Tuscaloosa Family Practice Residency at the University of Alabama. . . . The academic specialty of Family Medicine was still very new at the time and there were few seasoned role models within medical school ranks. Dr. Willard [dean of CCHS at the time] convinced Dr. Rutland in 1972 to give up two days per week from his practice in Fayette to teach family practice residents. He served as the Director of the Tuscaloosa Family Practice Residency from 1973–75. . . . Dr. Rutland is widely recognized for his central role in getting CCHS off to a good start.

Harold Reed, "Fayette County Medicine: A History of Quality Healthcare in Rural Alabama" (Rutland Papers, CHFM)

Besides seeing his patients, Rutland played a lot of different and important roles in his community. In 1960, he and his wife Nancy were voted Man and Woman of the Year in Fayette for devotion to their local community. As Harold Reed notes, Rutland was a local diving coach, worked as team doctor with two different high school football teams, was involved in his local church, and was a trustee of Fayette County High School.

In short, he had much of the talent, drive, and dedication the new specialty of family practice* wanted in its doctors when it got off the ground formally in 1969.

Enter the Specialty of Family Practice

The story of Richard Rutland is the hoped-for narrative of America's family practice. The new specialty of family practice in 1969 wanted to keep that iconic image of the generalist doctor—the image Richard Rutland represented. But it also wanted the new family doctor to be as good as if not better, intellectually and in pedigree, than physicians belonging to other specialties like internal medicine and surgery. It wanted to produce a new, improved version of the GP, at least on paper. One that would be accepted finally by the rest of the profession and have staying power with the public.

The idea was to try and have it all: a medical specialty filled with doctors that could think and treat holistically; practice relational medicine of the highest order; manage all aspects of patient care; devote themselves to their local communities and live within them for a long time; understand community-based and public health approaches to prevention and disease management; know in depth how to navigate services in those communities; *and* possess a wide breadth of clinical knowledge, decision-making expertise, and patient care experience compared to other doctors. Doctors who understood how to refer patients to specialists but who could keep as much in house as possible to promote comprehensive, cost-effective care delivery.

Family practice wanted to produce thousands of intellectually supercharged, well-trained, personable, crusader-type Richard Rutlands who would work not only in small towns in rural America but in big cities like New York and in the ever-expanding middle-class suburban com-

---

* The terms *family medicine* and *family practice* will be used interchangeably throughout the book. Purists of course will note that the term *family practice* was the official moniker given to the field at the start. But the certification board is called the Advisory Board of Family Medicine and the term *family medicine* has always been used to refer to both the content and intellectual scope of the specialty.

munities of the 1970s. Doctors who would make patients remember the old generalist but at the same time thank their lucky stars for this new breed of family physician before them, who could take charge of their care. There was a strong sense among early leaders in the movement that the traditional form of general practitioner (GP) was already dead, and in terms of medical student interest and the larger profession they were right. Medical students were not interested in becoming GPs during the 1960s, even though the demand for primary care was growing exponentially with the creation of Medicaid and Medicare. The medical profession was calling for the GP to be replaced with a new kind of doctor who could provide comprehensive care (Millis 1966). The idea was to seize the moment with a new type of comprehensive physician. One mass-produced through a new, impressive training regimen and a larger institutional structure that brought consistency and rigor to the process of educating family doctors.

The beginning of a formal family practice specialty in America started with a bang. The late 1960s, a time of social unrest and upheaval in America, provided the right context in which this new uber-brand of family doctor could spawn and flourish. The reimagined field of family medicine brought great hope for a return to generalist medicine in the United States. Only this time, it would be different. Building its training and socialization structures to compete for students' attention with other growing surgical and primary care specialties like internal medicine and positioning itself as part of the "counterculture" fighting to transform American life in the decades of the 1960s and 1970s, family practice would succeed where the specialty of general practice had failed.

It would legitimize itself by looking like other specialties, at least in form if not fully in substance. There would be a three-year training period, a formal oversight board approved by the medical profession at large, embedding of its teaching professionals and training programs in academic medical centers, and formal certification and recertification through standardized exams made for a specialty that could claim the moral high ground in relation to its purpose and be accepted for its intellectual rigor. It would require a rebranding campaign built in part on imitation and flattery of the way other clinical specialties trained their members.

Family practice would also succeed by identifying itself as part of the counterculture movement arising in American society during the late 1960s and 1970s (Stephens 1979). It would be a medical specialty committed to community medicine, advocacy, and making society better—not one narrowly fixated on individual patient care. It would contain a good portion of doctors who could be persistent in the influence they sought to exert on their surroundings. It would serve a collective purpose beyond the notion of science-based, ivory-tower medicine. It would exist for the collective pursuit of a greater good. As G. Gayle Stephens, perhaps family practice's greatest thought leader, noted a decade after the specialty's founding:

> Family practice, more or less knowingly, has been deeply involved in social reform and . . . we owe a great deal of our success to that. Clearly, we have been on the side of change in American life. We have identified ourselves with certain minorities and minority positions. We have been counter to many of the dominant forces in society. In some respects at least we belong to the counterculture. . . . Family physicians, accustomed to being "outsiders," were willing to take on, in a self-conscious way, the reform spirit of the 1960s and to identify themselves with issues that have deep roots in American history: the preservation of rural life, humane values, consumerism, and the rights of women. (Stephens 1989, p. 108)

A Specialty Fallen Short and a Primary Care Crisis

To many observers' eyes, though, the reality of family practice's existence over time has not met the ambitious dream its intellectuals and forebearers imagined. Doing primary care medicine right remains perhaps the most difficult job in health care. Why? For starters, there are too many people who have real illnesses and complex conditions. Too many with mental health problems and life circumstances stacked against them that affect their health but that a family doctor cannot do much to improve. That said, in most parts of the United States, there are many people walking around town who could benefit from having a single doctor get to know them, manage their care needs, and simply listen to them when they need it. Many more than in Richard Rutland's day. But there are not enough family doctors to do this, and the doctors left are overwhelmed as a result. Second, most family doctors now work as employees for larger health care corporations that control what they do and how they do it. Even for those family doctors willing to try and fulfill the comprehensive role, they must deal with employers who dictate the terms of how they will fill that role. Third, many family doctors have grown used to working nine-to-five as a physician, and they value their work-life balance and going home at night free of the need to be on call for patients.

There are high workloads and job dissatisfaction for many family doctors these days. But so what? Why should we feel sorry for family doctors who are still very well compensated for what they do compared to others and who still maintain a lot of autonomy over their work? Who have the kind of status and prestige most of us only dream about? Why should we care? Because health care is central to our lives. There is nothing perhaps more important to keeping us happy and productive, and living a long time, than our health care. And family doctors, of all the doctors in existence, are most responsible and able to keep us healthy (Basu et al. 2019). If they can be true generalists; if they are allowed to perform their role to at least some level of what Richard Rutland could do; if they can establish long-term relationships and trust with each of us; if they want to get up and do this kind of work each day, fulfilled and happy to be doing it, it is irrelevant how much they are paid when their value to us is this great. What matters is if they can do the work and be the professional needed to deliver the right kind of health care to us.

The dream of generalist doctors loyal to patients and vice versa remains elusive. The health care system provides a difficult proving ground for doing comprehensive medicine. It provides severe bureaucratic constraints related to measuring quality, justifying appropriate reimbursement for primary care service, using time-intensive electronic medical records, and taking care of patients personally. It has taken control away from the doctor by making most of them salaried employees. As employees of larger health corporations and systems, these doctors have a harder time advocating for themselves and their patients. They cannot easily oversee and secure their patients' health information, which hinders their ability to develop relationships with patients. Their work gets narrowed by organizations interested in efficiency and having family doctors see as many patients as possible in the office.

Owning a family practice office has grown untenable for the individual doctor, making salaried employment the only viable career choice. Once made employees, many family doctors see less personal value for making the major career and lifestyle sacrifices necessary to be a Richard Rutland–type healer. They diversify their job choices and pursue several different opportunities, few of which keep them close to being the generalist doctor taking care of the same patients over time in some small corner of America. They splinter as a collective group, becoming unable to band together and assert their common interests easily. This places them even more at the mercy of health systems and corporate employers who take charge in defining the doctor's job, their compensation, and, ultimately, their interactions with patients.

Family practice has accomplished some important things for American health care, and for itself. It helped bring health care services to increasing numbers of patients as public programs like Medicare and Medicaid were expanding. It normalized to some extent a greater focus on keeping people healthier through better chronic disease management, a focus on prevention, and regular trips to visit the doctor. It helped in raising to prominence aspects of public health such as screening for various diseases, vaccinations, and the role social determinants play in our health. It gave many people a focal point for having their care coordinated and managed within a fragmented delivery system. It kept the notion of the generalist doctor alive.

Yet on the ground and over time it has fallen far shorter in transforming our health care system. Yes, one can still find some family doctors doing comprehensive medicine in inner-city community health centers and rural-based primary care offices. Some of these doctors do the kinds of things Richard Rutland did; they are part of the communities they serve, and they have very strong relationships with many of their patients. But those overall numbers of doctors remain small and stagnant, and they are increasingly subject to the oversight of corporate-owned health systems that see primary care medicine as a feeder for more expensive care delivery. This happens increasingly in rural areas as well given the onslaught of health care mergers and acquisitions across the country, and the reality is that only the large health care corporation can provide the resources and scale needed to have accessible care in these geographic areas.

The specialty of family practice has not created the vast army of full-spectrum, highly trained generalists it first imagined would be everywhere throughout the United States. Most US medical students remain unconvinced, like they were about general practice in the 1960s, and they opt instead for other specialties, consistently leaving half or more of family physician residency positions vacant year after year that are then filled with graduates of non-US medical schools (National Resident Matching Program 2019). Judging from the current compensation of family doctors relative to other specialties, it has also not convinced the American public, policy makers, or insurers that its brand of physician is the best and should be higher paid (Doximity 2019). Reimbursement for primary care services lags behind what procedure-based specialties recoup for their services, despite the lip service paid by policy makers and third-party payers.

Patients increasingly question, in our corporatized, technologically driven delivery system, what it is that such doctors can do for them that merits greater inconvenience in their lives, such as waiting days or months for a family physician office appointment (Merritt Hawkins 2017). Increasingly, most people under the age of 30 have never had a family doctor they could call their own (Boodman 2018). Policy makers and industry stakeholders like hospitals and pharmacy chains push disruptive innovations that undermine getting care in the family physician's office, such as opening up retail health clinics and urgent care centers, creating smartphone-based virtual care, and giving a wider scope of practice to non-physician providers like nurse practitioners. All of this furthers a cheaper, non-physician-centric version of primary care medicine among the public and insurers (Griggs 2019; Hoff 2017; Landi 2019).

Those who are or will soon be family doctors make increasingly pragmatic and short-term career choices that lead them further away from the original family medicine ideal described above. They find themselves focusing on career "survival" or career "sustainability" to pay back immense amounts of debt, avoid burnout, have a richer non-work lifestyle, give their lives greater flexibility to do other things, and avoid taking on too much administrative work (American Academy of Family Physicians 2019; Hoff 2010; Medscape 2018). Many say in a perfect world they would want to be family doctors in the ideal sense. But they acknowledge that to do it right intimidates them—demanding more of their time, energy, employment stability, and brain power, even at the risk of lower pay and greater personal hassle for doing it.

A lot of the young family doctors are trained without getting connected to the world of the generalist family physician working out in the community. They do not get to see firsthand the joy of generalist work, of having longitudinal relationships with patients, of contributing to the health of their community. They train mostly in hospitals and inpatient settings, doing work that is not generalist in nature. They see patients in hospital clinics that are not representative of the kinds of patients they would have in a community practice; clinic patients that are sicker, often more noncompliant, and more transitory. This often gives a less than positive image of the generalist role and makes the myriad of work duties involved in managing a patient's care needs seem onerous and not worth the effort.

Increasing numbers of older family doctors retire earlier than they want, go part-time, or leave direct patient care for other work (Physicians Foundation 2018). Younger ones also work part-time more, or become hospitalists doing inpatient medicine rather than the work of disease prevention and keeping people healthy. They perform shift work with unknown patients in urgent care centers and other settings and work rigidly set schedules as paid employees for large delivery systems where the patients are not theirs but rather belong to the health care corporation (Frank et al. 2019; Medscape 2018).

The story of family practice in America is one of a prolonged identity crisis: of lofty and stubbornly held ideals that have fallen short; of an inability to adapt in sensible ways that make patients see the value;

of overconfidence about its presumed counterculture mission and how it could be achieved, but which has not been supported by increased boots on the ground turning to it as their career choice; of significant moments of incremental progress almost always undermined by an inhospitable health care system. It is a story about how a large and important institution that has always wanted to create a certain type of doctor, and which labels itself implicitly as a nobler undertaking than other medical specialties, has paid less attention to how its own members think and feel about their work and the full range of what its patients want from their health care.

The specialty of family practice seems to know less about what its members are experiencing in the real world of health care, for if it did, one would hope it would use all its collective energy to try and change that world now, including the ways its members must take career matters into their own hands, which makes them more attuned to short-term personal survival than enacting the family physician role in a different way. The specialty of family practice continues to seek the path of acceptance from other medical specialties, payers, and the public by following the same playbook as those other specialties. It still imitates them rather than trying to establish itself as something very different. It retains a meaningful inferiority complex when looking at itself alongside the rest of the medical profession.

This book examines what happens to an overly hyped medical specialty and its doctors when a hostile health care system continues to turn its back on the ideal of the generalist physician and the goals of relational medicine. We all should care about this story, because without a large group of family doctors able to practice comprehensive primary care, our health suffers. Without generalist doctors who know something about us, who we trust and can listen to, and who can coordinate all our health care needs, we are set adrift into a system that does not care about us. We are left to fend for ourselves, trying to figure out on our own when we need to get care, what clinical advice to listen to, and how to lead healthier lives. Without a strong generalist physician contingent, health care becomes just another transactional service delivery system in our lives. A system which convinces us that speed, convenience, and no-frills service are better than long-term relationships with a doctor that include trust, respect, compassion, and empathy.

This important story unfolds in two interrelated ways. First, through the voices of those professionals, young and old, who have chosen or are now choosing to be family doctors. These individuals, some who became family physicians in the 1970s and 1980s and others in or just out of family medicine residency, answer similar questions about the hoped-for and everyday fulfillment of their expectations and identities as generalists. They share their career thinking and choices, the work they have done or do and how it has shaped them as physicians, and the feelings they have toward their craft, specialty, and the family doctor ideal. They share their struggles. They provide valuable insight into why they became doctors, why they chose family medicine, and the various bargains they make, like all workers, to achieve some semblance of career satisfaction and meaning for themselves in addition to financial security and a less stressful way of life.

Some of these bargains have not been good for the specialty's long-term health. They are not the bargains Richard Rutland had to consider or make. They have negatively affected and continue to undermine the long-term health of the family medicine specialty, and in the process, they have weakened our primary care system and the goal of health care as a humane endeavor. They have balkanized the specialty, making its members unable to collectively advocate for themselves in ways that might force their employers to serve their interests, rather than the other way around. They have also put others between family doctors and their patients, making it harder to develop the kinds of relationships that would make the public more aware of and loyal to the family doctor ideal.

What this story shows clearly is how patients lose out when family doctors end up having to take matters into their own hands. It shows how increasing cynicism and career angst among family doctors influences their attitudes and behaviors toward their craft in ways that weaken the potential for relational excellence with patients and makes the notion of generalist doctors more a dream than reality. To do primary care right requires doctors deeply committed to their patients, and it requires the time and energy necessary to weather the bureaucracy and uncertainties the modern health care system throws at them every day. But family doctors are human beings as well. What those interviewed here show is that theirs is a mighty struggle to reconcile personal self-interest and career happiness with the necessary sacrifices of being a contemporary generalist physician.

Older family doctors talk about what they did career-wise and how they did it, and how they feel about it now. Younger family doctors and medical students going into family medicine discuss what they want to do in their careers, the reasons why, and if they think they will be happy doing it. The career experiences, intents, and hopes of these family doctors, young and old, have much to say about where family medicine is, where it wanted to be, why it is not there yet, and where it is going. Interwoven through these voices is a critical analysis of the early evolution of the family practice specialty—that is, the events, rhetoric, and strategic decision making that shaped how this medical field would evolve over the next fifty years. That early evolution determined how the specialty would ultimately position itself in the larger health system and medical profession over the past half century, and how individual family doctors would come to see themselves and their careers. It has determined in part the level of personal sacrifice today's family doctors are willing to make in moving toward the generalist ideal.

The story of early family practice evolution and the current career experiences of its doctors is a story that informs our understanding about the future prospects for our most important kind of patient care, *primary care*, which for a long time many have believed performs better when physicians deliver it, and when it is done in a way that focuses on prevention that treats people in a holistic and continuous manner. The disruption occurring in our primary care system at present, much of it not involving an embrace of the family physician model, suggests that the specialty and its doctors face an uphill battle in promoting a relational, physician-centric version of primary care for the future.

There are many hospitals, insurers, venture capitalists, and tech companies that right now do not believe family doctors should or need to be at the center of most primary care of the future (Rand 2016). Given this emerging united front of adversaries, many of them with deep pockets, we need to know how prepared mentally, emotionally, experientially, and skills-wise family doctors are to engage in this fight for the soul of a major segment of American health care. If they are not ready, it will be difficult for family doctors to remain at the forefront of primary care transformation, and they won't be able to fulfill its ideal. This would mean a very different kind of health care system in our lives. One potentially without a highly skilled autonomous professional as our point person. Instead, the corporation with its primary care franchises, slick marketing campaigns, data trove of patient information, and wealth of analytics tools will be serving in that role. Primary care is the canary in the coal mine for seeing the type of patient care we may have in America in the future.

The story of how family doctors and their specialty are evolving also speaks to the larger story of how medicine is changing rapidly from the inside out, after years of being squeezed by social, political, technological, and economic forces questioning its power and demanding it change. The American medical profession is indeed adapting, that much is true, but how and who is driving such adaptation remain open questions; and what that adaptation looks like on the ground is still relatively unknown. The story here suggests that at least one specialty and its doctors are taking matters too much into their own hands. This may not be good for either them or their profession over time. It may play right into the hands of those stakeholders who wish to see health care controlled less by the professional and more by the corporation.

Through this combined macro- and micro-level analysis, I hope to draw some important conclusions about the present and future of this particular professional specialty; a specialty that on a theoretical level embodies many of the chief features that define a just, humane, and patient-centric health care system. Whether such a system is possible or realistic, given what has already happened to our health care system over time, is a fair question. Yet the time is now to determine if family physicians and their specialty can help spearhead the fight toward this elusive goal. Otherwise, the Richard Rutlands of the world and what they have stood for will stay relegated to the history books. Quaint museum pieces of a once-thought possible reality that never thrived on a grand enough scale to transform how we think about our health care or our lives.

Dear Dr. Rutland,

We will always remember and be thankful for your dedication and your kind consideration and compassion during our time of need, especially in taking care of Pearl over the years. You were always able to make it well. Just a pat on the back from you and a few kind words, was more effective than medicine. . . .

    We love & cherish you,

    James O. & Minnie P.

    Patient letter to Dr. Rutland upon his retirement, 1997 (Rutland Papers, Center for the History of Family Medicine [CHFM])

TWO

Poor Soil for Growing Generalists

Family Doctors versus the Health System

WHEN I WORKED in primary care as an administrator back in the late 1980s, I heard the same complaint from the family doctors with whom I worked as I do now from those that I interview for my research— primary care medicine is not paid for in the United States anywhere commensurate with its value to patients. When I helped to run an insurance billing department for a primary care office thirty years ago, I saw firsthand how much lower the payments were for services meant to keep people from getting sick compared to payment for services that relied on waiting for people to get sick. Not much has changed in 2021. There is the rhetoric that primary care and prevention matter much more now to insurance companies, hospitals, and doctors' offices. Sure, maybe in a few areas like chronic disease management where primary care medicine and family doctors have been asked to do more for patients. But that has not created a financial windfall for primary care, and what it asks of family doctors is very much responsible for how joyless some of their patient care work has become. For the most part, high-cost specialty medicine still dominates the health care system and still receives the bulk of the insurance payments. It is responsible for keeping hospitals profitable and specialist doctors well paid and in control.

The specialty of family medicine has always existed within the context of an unsupportive American health care system that underemphasizes primary care, where service is fragmented and procedural medicine is favored, and that waits until people get sick to interact with them and is ever more corporatized (Starr 1982). It is a care delivery system long built on capitalist ideals. One defined by a supply side which pushes the prevailing narrative that health care is not a fundamental individual right, but rather a market in which buyers and sellers come together to transact business that benefits both sides (Rosenthal 2018). Despite the advent of Medicare and Medicaid in the 1960s, and the Affordable Care Act in 2010, health care in America since the 1970s has been mostly about providing big ticket items to an unhealthy, largely uninformed group of patients. That is where the money has always been for hospitals and specialists. This profit motive has produced a care delivery system in which monopolistic behavior and service fragmentation abound, politicians serve powerful industry stakeholders in biased ways, growth is valued above all else, and patients are left mostly out of the equation (Rosenthal 2018).

To create such a cold-blooded system takes time. It has not happened overnight. Neither will it be fixed overnight. Such a system is no friend to either family medicine or primary care. In fact, such a system views primary care as an attractive nuisance, useful for capturing patients in more expensive systems of care and getting them efficiently to higher-cost services (Hoff 2017). A loss leader to get patients to the expensive stuff. The American health care system has for decades been less enthusiastic to the idea of a generalist doctor managing patients' care holistically and with a high level of relational excellence. It has financially undervalued primary care in all its forms. It has allowed the job of a family doctor to become saddled with administrative chores and bureaucratic requirements. It has made family doctors buy into one new initiative after another, overpromising how these initiatives would help primary care while under delivering. In many ways, it has treated family doctors like the generalists of old they replaced—as lower-valued and lower-paid parts of American medicine.

The Financial Undervaluing of Primary Care

All things hostile to family medicine in the American health care system start with reimbursement. And reimbursement has not been kind to family medicine and primary care delivery over the years. In terms of receiving adequate payment for its services, primary care medicine has always been the ugly stepchild of American health care. In other countries like Canada and the United Kingdom, primary care medicine and its doctors remain the centerpiece of care delivery and receive a significant bulk of the resources, but in the United States it has not been that way since World War II (Starr 1982). Continued advances in medical technology, the rise of hospitals and specialists, and an ambivalent public have been steady negative influences on primary care's viability.

Aiding these developments beginning in post–World War II America was the increased availability of private insurance for many Americans, usually paid by employers. Before insurance, generalist doctors dealt in a cash-only business, charging patients fixed fees for different types of services. Their system of billing was perhaps less egalitarian in giving everyone the chance to obtain their services, but it was within physicians' control and fully transparent. Patients knew how much a service would cost, and they could assess whether it was worth the cost to have it performed, at least from their personal perspective. Doctors, almost all of whom owned their practices, could in theory better manage their revenue and expenses, altering their prices in relation to how much time and other resources were put into the service provided. Such a payment system helped to keep generalist medicine an economically viable endeavor in which a single doctor could be involved as an owner. One might not get wealthy, but you could earn a good living, control the economics of your practice, and do the kind of medicine that you wanted with your patients.

Then insurance came along (see Starr 1982). Private insurance separated patients from the costs of various forms of care, making specialty medicine an attractive option with fewer financial risks associated with it. While other countries like Canada and the United Kingdom insured most of their populations through government-run programs that had spending caps and placed primary care medicine at the center of care delivery, the United States pursued its insurance expansion in a different way, focused for decades on fee-for-service reimbursement and providing "usual and customary" payments to doctors based largely on what the latter wanted to charge for their services (Ortiz-Ospina and Roser 2019).

Insurance in American health care undercut the economic rewards of primary care medicine for family doctors because it biased payments toward procedures and specialists. It prevented patients from understanding "value" when it came to diagnosis or treatment and many no longer needed to worry about how much a health service cost. The fee-for-service payment system over time paid out more bills at a higher rate for specialists than for primary care doctors, because the usual and customary fees were set by specialists themselves, with little questioning of how they came up with their fees (Berenson and Rich 2010).

Good primary care medicine is slower to do than most procedural work. It does not align well with procedural medicine that can be done in an assembly-line fashion, generating a higher volume of overall fees in the process. Family medicine or primary care involves something called "evaluation and management services," which in essence is time the family doctor spends on interviewing the patient, asking questions, getting to know patients, and managing a wide swath of clinical complaints and treatments for some. Attempting to be someone's "comprehensive doctor" and "care manager" means a lot of these types of tasks and activities. Many of these tasks and activities simply have not been as highly valued dollar-wise by insurers. But they are critical to a close-knit doctor-patient relationship. Just ask Dr. Richard Rutland and his patients.

March 25, 1997

Dear Dr. Rutland:

As a doctor, you have always been a great inspiration to me. Just like the mail carrier you are there rain, sleet, snow, or sunshine, with a great smile for your patients. You're always friendly, you get to know your patients' wants, needs, and their pains as you try to help accommodate them. You always try to give your patient your best and that is what a great doctor should do for his patients. . . . You're just like a member of the family.

Your friend and patient, Maurice.

Patient letter to Dr. Rutland upon his retirement, 1997 (Rutland Papers, CHFM)

Whereas specialists are niche providers focused on treating single diagnoses and body parts, family doctors in theory are practicing medicine focused on prevention, disease management, behavioral health, and family care. They rely on getting to know their patients' preferences, needs, and wants to deliver this type of medicine effectively. They must get patients to trust and listen to them. Primary care medicine takes more time as a result. It also has a longer trajectory to seeing the end results because it is more uncertain and complicated for many patients, involves a lot of cognitive work on the part of the doctor, and often has delayed time frames for seeing good outcomes. As a result of these realities, most primary care services are also difficult to price accurately. Add to this the idea that in many geographic areas there have been fewer proceduralists than primary care doctors, with the former often banding together in large practices to exert power over the insurance companies and hospitals, and reimbursement has favored specialty care.

Resource-Based Relative Value Scale, Managed Care, and Other False Payment Promises for Family Doctors

Things did not get better for primary care reimbursement in the 1990s. Two developments on the reimbursement front, presumed initially to help level the payment playing field for family doctors, had unintended consequences that continued to hurt family doctors, particularly those who owned their own offices. The first development, the Resource-Based Relative Value Scale (RBRVS), came along in 1992, led by Medicare (American Medical Association 2020a). The RBRVS was a payment formula meant to equalize the reimbursement value placed on procedures versus those evaluation and management services family doctors spent most of their time on (Bodenheimer et al. 2007).

By pricing services according to how long they took, for example, and in consideration of the full scope of resources that went into them, the idea was that office-based primary care medicine, which in its purest form contained a lot of complex interactions and visits with patients, and a lot of physician time, should earn higher reimbursements from third-party payers. The calculations that went into the Relative Value Unit numbers, attached to each service and procedure, were determined by a Relative Value Scale Update Committee, a panel of two dozen representatives across the different specialties who met regularly to hammer out which services and procedures were worth how much (American Medical Association 2020b).

Why anyone who invented the RBRVS payment system would think that a committee composed of approximately 90 percent specialists and 10 percent primary care doctors would help equalize payment for primary care services with specialist services is a mystery likely never to be solved. Suffice it to say, reimbursement under this system remained heavily tilted toward paying more for procedural versus primary care medicine. Worse, it did nothing to discourage the do-more-get-more reality that fee-for-service medicine promoted among specialists. In a system where no one demanded which type of doctor a patient needed to see, specialists continued to thrive over family doctors. They had the better brand with patients (Hoff 2017).

Patients with good insurance, usually from their employers, did not need to worry about paying more to see specialists, because insurers usually paid without needing primary care doctors to sign off on it, or even see the patient first. Under a fee-for-service system, the more specialists did, the more reimbursement they got. All of this took valuable dollars away from family doctors who were increasingly denied opportunities to help patients decide whether those high-cost specialist visits and procedural work were always necessary. They were also denied opportunities to perform some of this care for patients, which led to a narrower scope of work for the family doctor, which then fed into a devaluing of that doctor. This devaluing could be seen in the lower salaries of primary care compared to other specialist doctors and in the growing salary divide over time. For example, in 1975 the average net income for general practitioners was $44,000 compared to $61,000 for general surgeons. By 1985, the net income for general surgeons was approximately $111,000 compared to $73,000 for general practitioners (Langenbrunner et al. 1988).

How these payment realities impacted patients was fewer medical students choosing to become family doctors and instead choosing higher-paying specialties. It furthered a primary care physician shortage in many parts of the United States, resulting in patients who could not easily access any type of health care in their communities, since specialists were harder to find in rural areas and inner cities. It made trying to build a Richard Rutland–type office in one's community a very difficult and risky thing to do for family doctors. It also demoralized many generalist physicians who were being asked to go the extra mile in building long-term relationships with growing numbers of patients.

In the 1990s, a well-intended but misguided attempt to change this dysfunctional, anti–primary care delivery system came along in the form of "managed care." It is apparent now that no one then understood that the main problem with this approach started with its name, and family doctors suffered because of that name. While countries like the United Kingdom and Canada manage care all the time, and their citizens grow used to it in return for everyone having universal insurance coverage, in the United States calling anything *managed* can invoke a visceral reaction from the public, few of whom likes to be told what types of choices they can make in their daily lives. The backbone of the managed care approach consisted of "physician gatekeeping" and "capitation payment" (Friedman 1996), both of which were doomed from the start. Doomed because eventually both would be perceived by patients for what they inevitably were, attempts by insurers to control how much care people received. Doomed because they smeared family doctors with the same broad brush used to label insurance companies as *care rationers*. Once a group of doctors gets associated with the insurance side of the industry, it becomes that much harder for the public to like them.

The entire managed care approach rested on something called *capitation*. Capitation was a payment system in which doctors, but in this case primary care doctors, received "per member, per month" dollars in return for: (a) those doctors serving as the gatekeepers overseeing each individual patient's use of health care services; and (b) providing basic preventive services designed to keep their patients healthier, thereby lowering the downstream costs of patients having to visit specialists after they had gotten sick (Berwick 1996). Capitation was also known as *prospective payment* in the sense that it was a payment system meant to incentivize family doctors to behave more conservatively (with respect to referring patients to specialty care or using expensive testing) and proactively (with respect to engaging the patient in prevention) by giving them payment for their time and work up front. As a form of prospective payment, capitation was designed to right the wrongs associated with fee-for-service medicine, that do-more-get-more system allowing patients to bypass their family doctors and go directly to specialists. Capitation was a payment system that, in theory, meant to elevate the role of the family doctor to premier status in the health care system.

Only it did not turn out that way. First, no one liked any physician, family doctor or otherwise, strictly controlling their care options, so patients in capitated systems experienced greater dissatisfaction (Kerr et al. 1999). Even if it made sense from a system perspective, the branding of gatekeeping soon became one of rationed care. This placed the family doctor increasingly at odds with their patients. In addition, while the concept of paying family doctors in advance for providing preventive services to their patients, and keeping them healthier, sounded great, in practice it was a logistical nightmare for doctors and patients. Getting patients to proactively come into the office for a preventive visit, or to engage in self-management at home, became more difficult than imagined. American patients were schooled to visit doctors and think about their health care when they were sick, not when they were healthy, so it is not like all patients would come in for regular preventive care on their own, adding to the burden on family doctors to get their patients into the office. Busy family doctors with already full visit schedules and lots of administrative work to do found it easy to forget about giving what could be a lot of time to prevention activities, and the dollars allotted for them through capitation often turned out to be grossly insufficient to make ends meet (Yarnall et al. 2012).

Capitation was also a payment approach that gave birth to the modern quality movement—where every single activity is measured and family doctors have become record keepers for insurance companies and Medicare to show that they are trying to keep patients healthy (Hoff 2017). Family doctors must now pay for a lot of expensive infrastructure, such as electronic health records, to comply with modern quality-reporting requirements (Casalino et al. 2016). This expense began with managed care and capitation in the early 1990s, and it is one reason why fewer family doctors own their businesses and more become salaried employees whose employers pay for the infrastructure, not them (Kane 2019). Electronic health records and the added workload associated with using them has probably lent more to the reason why so many family doctors are burned out and dissatisfied than any other single feature of the modern medical workplace (Shanafelt et al. 2015).

This added workload is not the kind of extra work Richard Rutland performed. Whereas Rutland's work involved direct patient care, seeing a patient in the hospital in the evening or a patient in the emergency room on the weekend for example, or doing a house call outside of normal office hours, the family doctor's added work under managed care and through today involves heavy doses of administrative duties, that is, completing paperwork for insurance companies, completing documentation to satisfy various quality metrics, and getting authorizations for needed services, referrals to other doctors, and medications.

For family doctors, there was one more innovation during the first decade of the twenty-first century intended to place their roles as comprehensive physicians into greater prominence in the system. The main problem was that in the end, this innovation, called the *patient-centered medical home* (PCMH), also increased the family doctor's workload without increasing their reimbursement meaningfully, if at all (Osborn et al. 2015). The PCMH model, like prior efforts that sounded great on paper for family doctors, brought with it big expectations for better and more proactive chronic disease care, care for senior populations, and holistic care across an individual's life span.

Family doctors would become the "medical home" for their patients, implying that patients would seek them out before getting care in other parts of the system. This term *medical home* was the hook that attracted family doctors to it initially. But without much new money injected into the primary care system, family doctors weren't able to earn more for this added work, nor were they able to invest in the additional practice resources required to do "medical home care" right (National Committee for Quality Assurance 2019). The PCMH has not been the boon to family medicine once thought, nor has it repositioned primary care at the center of health care delivery in the United States. For instance, the added reimbursement for converting one's practice into a medical home has not been sufficient for many primary care doctors given the greater time and resources needed to comply with the model's requirements (Basu et al. 2016).

At present, the primary care reimbursement scene for family doctors to practice full-spectrum, holistic medicine still looks no better. Every few years it seems new payment models are tried, each offered as "revolutionary" for the field of primary care. But most never scale up beyond smaller, localized pilot initiatives. Others seem to bring as much heartache to the work of a family doctor as they do additional dollars—if they bring any new dollars at all. These include Accountable Care Organizations (ACOs) that are supposed to get hospitals and specialists to focus more on keeping certain groups of patients healthy and utilization lower, favoring primary care delivery; bundled payment systems intended to incentivize different care delivery stakeholders to collaborate and use primary care to lower the overall costs of care; and pay-for-performance programs, emanating from big payers like Medicare, that offer the potential for enhanced reimbursement to family doctors if they practice high-quality, efficient medicine. None of these initiatives have been shown to be the magic bullet saving primary care from the depths of low prestige and low compensation.

That said, more doctors than ever before participate in these new models of care that seek to redesign how physicians are paid. Family physicians are increasingly forced into unproven payment models on the promise that their reimbursements may increase (Rama 2018). In a 2018 survey of almost 9,000 physicians across the United States, 55 percent of primary care doctors said that they participated in value-based payment models such as ACOs or bundled payments, and 70 percent of primary care doctors had upwards of 30 percent of their total compensation tied to the quality and efficiency metrics defining such payment models. That said, many of these doctors also think that being paid in these new ways has not improved the quality or cost effectiveness of their work (Physicians Foundation 2018).

The main point is this—for the longest time, the field of primary care has been reimbursed poorly compared to other medical specialties (Neumann et al. 2019). This reality has not changed, with family doctors in 2020 facing largely the same insufficient reimbursement landscape for their services as they did in 2015, 2010, and 2000. It has not changed for two main reasons: (a) what gets asked of family doctors in return for potentially earning more at each of these time points is too ambitious or downright onerous and impossible to fulfill given their heavy patient workloads and inefficient ways their practices are designed; and (b) because ultimately the new dollars that are injected into the primary care system are not close to adequate to either fairly compensate for these new activities or motivate family doctors to make other changes that could accommodate those activities. These payment innovations also ironically demotivate the family doctor from providing the kind of comprehensive care for patients that the specialty of family practice has always wanted its members to provide. Finally, looming over this payment fiasco is the rise of an entire monitoring infrastructure that has taken control away from family doctors and undercut the focus on relational excellence in primary care (Hoff 2017).

Many have argued that such reimbursement disparity with specialty care is the main reason primary care in the United States has withered on the vine. That may be partially true. But it has not been the only factor. Blaming reimbursement oversimplifies the complete story of family medicine's inability to gain full traction in American health care. This underinvestment in primary care is not just a US phenomenon; many government-funded systems, like the United Kingdom's and Canada's, now cut primary care budgets regularly, at the same time they want family doctors and the field of primary care to do more (Robertson et al. 2014). In fact, the past several decades have seen most industrialized nations look to their primary care systems in a paradoxical way—as the solution to lowering costs and improving quality in patient care, while at the same time making them ground zero in the health services underinvestment trend.

This pits a specialty like family practice, built ideally on time-consuming activities, like care coordination and management, evaluation and management services, and building long-term relationships with patients, at odds with the system itself. It also keeps the specialty relegated to a second-class citizen status in comparison with procedurally oriented specialties among insurers, hospital systems, patients, and policy makers. After all, if you were asked which meal you thought was higher quality and better tasting, the one that cost $100 a plate or the one that cost $10 a plate, you would say the former almost every time, despite never having tasted either meal. The reimbursement environment around family medicine determines how it is thought about as a field of medicine, how it is pursued as a career option, and the sort of future that is in store for it. There is simply no way it cannot.

"Amazon Thinking," Technology, and "Pop-Up" Medical Care Dumbs Primary Care Down

Lower payments for primary care services; fewer family doctors who can make ends meet by owning practices, and so must become employees; the rise of large corporations controlling health care; paperwork demands making the job less than it could be; and fewer medical students wanting to enter the specialty because of what they see and hear about it are creating a perfect storm for disruptive innovation in primary care. A storm that has been brewing over the past two decades. Add to this a shortage of primary care doctors in many parts of the United States, and the opportunity arises for new players to enter the scene. This disruption is characterized by limiting the use of high-cost family doctors and using cheaper non-physician labor instead; overhyping technological solutions and standardization for "better" care delivery; seeing the patient as a "consumer" wanting convenience over everything else; and downplaying the importance of human-based, relational care excellence.

Primary care is first and foremost ground zero for disruption through "Amazon thinking" (see Hoff 2017). No doubt, this progressive fracturing and dumbing down of primary care service delivery through cheaper, quicker, and more episodic touch points for patients is also the result of the increased demand for primary care brought on by insurance expansion under the Affordable Care Act. In many parts of the United States, wait times to see primary care doctors are excessive (Merritt Hawkins 2017), and Amazon thinking is designed in part to provide a lower-cost, accessible platform for basic primary care delivery (Farr 2018). The physician-centric primary care system has not had adequate supply to meet demand for some time now.

Nothing presents a greater threat to the specialty of family medicine, its doctors, and its goals of holistic, highly relational patient care than the application of efficiency-oriented business thinking and retail tactics, honed in other industries, to the delivery of primary care services. Why is this thinking such a threat? First, it diminishes the importance of the highly paid physician-expert in patient care, largely because that physician is the most expensive, least controllable input into the primary care production process. It is hard to control and reduce the cost of a given production flow when you cannot manipulate the highest-cost input in that flow. Newer primary care players such as Amazon, Apple, CVS Health, Walmart, and Walgreens do not want to employ family doctors. They do not want to have to depend on them either. Instead, their staffing focus is on cheaper and less skilled non-physician personnel such as nurse practitioners, physician assistants, registered nurses, and medical assistants (Tosto 2019).

The use of non-physician labor to deliver primary care has facilitated the increasing rise of "pop-up" offices in many communities that use nurse practitioners and physician assistants to deliver care (Rand 2016). As the United States experiences a shortage of primary care doctors, large health care companies like CVS Health and Walgreens maintain the scale and resources to create franchises that reimagine most primary care delivery as episodic visits and brief interactions. These emphasize convenience and the provision of basic services more than ongoing provider-patient relationships (Huckman 2019). These sites for primary care delivery are not based in physician-owned offices. Rather, they are owned and operated by big corporations (Japsen 2019). Retail-oriented forms of primary care delivery, like urgent care centers and minute clinics, emphasize transactional over relational excellence (see Hoff 2017).

The price point for each transaction remains lower compared to the traditional family doctor's office, which means doctors as the high-cost input are less welcome in the transaction, because that raises the overall price of the service. Things like convenience and timely access are meaningful goals for many patients who want primary care medicine today. But rather than being pursued as a complement to the relational care delivery patients also want and need, they now tend to become the primary focus for these new forms of primary care delivery (Hoff 2017).

A second related threat driving primary care disruption in a direction away from family doctors is the heavy use of technology in creating "dumbed-down" yet accessible forms of primary care medicine, soon to be done virtually on a wide scale through phones and smart devices like Amazon's Alexa. The pop-up primary care alternatives noted above rely heavily on using an integrated electronic health record system across their franchise locations that can standardize diagnostic and treatment protocols, for example, so that the non-physician providers delivering care in these settings all practice similarly.

In this way, the management of care and actual clinical decision making gets encoded into the computerized guideline and becomes the purview of the corporation, rather than the individual care provider. Patient data is "owned" by that corporation, and not the doctor or patient. The electronic health record (EHR), implemented now in every family doctor's workplace, is a disruptive technology that can undermine clinicians' feelings of autonomy, competence, and satisfaction (Kruse et al. 2016). As a technology designed in part to extract the knowledge of individual patients and their unique attributes from the family doctor's head and place it into a database that employers and others on the primary care team can easily access, the EHR sets the stage for other personnel to take over more of the family doctor's work and allows organizations to monitor what family doctors do and how they do it. Using artificial intelligence and lots of big data stored in electronic health records, many basic forms of primary care will likely be taken from the family doctor and given over to standardized computer algorithms for dispensing. For example, Babylon Health Care, one of these fledgling primary care disruptors, has invented chat bots that can rely on computerized algorithms to provide medical advice and some forms of clinical triage for patients, without a doctor ever having to step foot into the interaction with the patient (Babylon Health 2019).

As companies like Apple and Amazon gain control over these patient data through their cloud-based services, and various forms of primary care work are standardized in a recipe-like fashion to allow for that work to be broken into smaller pieces and apportioned to less skilled workers such as medical assistants and nurses, family doctors will lose some ability to perform the kinds of duties expected of them. In these ways, the EHR has been shown to de-skill family doctors in key ways that undercut their role as comprehensive physicians and care managers for their patients (Hoff 2011). It also has increased their everyday workloads greatly, forcing them to become data depositors for patients' insurance companies, entering quality metrics into the EHR to get reimbursed and generating mounds of patient information that requires their time and attention to sift through (Physicians Foundation 2018).

A key question is, how much of what family doctors now do will or can be replaced by this disruptive change? The smart money should be bet on the proposition that the forces pushing Amazon thinking and disruption into primary care will not stop anytime soon. The numbers of US medical students choosing family medicine remains flat, well short of what is required. Companies like Amazon, Apple, Walgreens, and CVS Health are not going away, as they seek to make primary care delivery a core part of their health care business strategy. These corporate behemoths are convinced there is low-hanging fruit to be had in squeezing profit out of services that can be made more standardized, lower cost, and highly transactional—chronic disease management, preventive and wellness care, and basic acute care. Some of the interest is in seeing this primary care service provision as a loss-leader, creating loyal customers who want to buy other health and non-health-related services and products from these companies (Japsen 2019). Smaller health care start-ups and the venture capital that supports them also see quick money in trying to help health care organizations use the vast sums of patient information they have collected to transform how primary care is done.

The family physician–driven model of primary care delivery is more expensive than these new forms of dumbed-down, transactional primary care. It requires more time, more inconvenience, and more face-to-face interaction with the patient, which is another reason why these alternative forms of primary care will continue to grow. It would not be so bad if they were a complement to highly relational, physician-centric primary care, but they are not presently. They seek to transform the way all of us think about health care generally, and primary care specifically.

For patients, Amazon thinking wants us to believe that physician interaction matters less in keeping us healthy. It wants us to believe that convenience and low cost matter as much if not more than the quality of the actual care delivered. It wants us to see our consumption of primary care services and products as one part of our larger consumption needs—right alongside the need for transportation, lodging, and a host of discretionary items we buy to make us happy. If successful in convincing us of this vision, Amazon thinking and the disruptive innovation associated with it presents as a serious threat to the future of family medicine and, more importantly, to the vision of healthy people and communities that family medicine stands for. It is yet another hostile force that an already-weakened family physician army must meet on the health care battlefield—a force bent on fully monetizing people's health by basing the health care services and products that are bought, sold, and profited from on transactional rather than relational excellence.

The Narrowing Scope of Family Doctor Work

A final big-picture reality creating a hostile environment for family doctors involves the continued narrowing of the family doctor's scope of practice. This narrowing is due to a combination of new and competing specialties, shifts in the personal values and work-related preferences of family physicians, the drive to maximize primary care reimbursement at the practice level, the shift of many services formerly done by family doctors to specialists, and the corporatization of primary care services that resigns many family physicians to predominantly office-based, outpatient work.

Make no mistake, the scope of work for family doctors has narrowed, with the percentage of family doctors performing activities involving maternity care, pediatrics, and women's health services declining over the past twenty years (Bazemore et al. 2012; Tong et al. 2012). This narrowing over time begets further narrowing because doctors who do less of something are likely to continue doing less of it given fears of malpractice and the accepted norm within medicine that doctors who do more of something get better at it and commit fewer errors.

One recent study comparing a sample of newly practicing family medicine residents trained in the late 1990s to those trained fifteen years later showed that residents trained later reported a much narrower scope of practice: 25 percent fewer residents were delivering babies, 32 percent fewer were doing inpatient medicine, 26 percent fewer were doing emergency care for their patients, 34 percent fewer were involved in intensive care medicine, 19 percent fewer were visiting their patients in nursing homes, and 28 percent fewer were doing any sort of assisted surgical care (Weidner and Chen 2019).

This is happening despite family residents trained later saying they felt they had been better prepared than the residents trained earlier to engage in these different types of clinical work. In addition, from the same study, the percentage of younger family doctors that performed sigmoidoscopy procedures (an example of a more complex procedure traditionally done by many family physicians years ago) was only 4 percent, compared to 42 percent of the older cohort. For other procedures such as intubation and placing central lines into patients, which also represent complex work, a higher percentage of family doctors trained in the late 1990s included these into their regular practice more often compared to those trained fifteen years later (Weidner and Chen 2019).

A 2015 study of almost 14,000 family doctors approached the issue of a narrower scope of practice for family doctors from a different angle, comparing brand new family doctors with ones who had been practicing longer. It surveyed groups of family practice board-exam recertifiers, that is, family doctors that were advanced in their careers (recertification in family practice is required every seven years), and certifiers, that is, family doctors just beginning their careers and taking the board exam for the first time. It found that early-career family doctors had an initially wider scope of practice, engaging in more activities such as prenatal care, obstetric care, and inpatient care. Meanwhile, the late-career recertifiers reported engaging in such activities significantly less (Coutinho et al. 2015). This study conveys that as a typical family doctor in the twenty-first century progresses in their career, what they do in their job begins departing from the ideal of the comprehensive physician, with their work growing less varied and full in scope.

Other specialties in organized medicine have sought out and claimed clinical turf that once belonged in the family practice domain. For example, in the 1970s, it was the new specialty of emergency medicine that took over care for all patients in hospital emergency rooms (ERs). There are now over 40,000 doctors specializing in emergency medicine. Prior to emergency medicine doctors, many family doctors assumed responsibility for providing care to their patients when the latter needed to visit an emergency room.

As time went on in the 1970s and 1980s, the economics of family doctors visiting their patients in ERs, during the night or, worse, when their own office practices were also open during the day, did not add up financially, as reimbursement for such emergency room visits lessened and the time expended for an ER visit of a single patient took the place of multiple in-office visits that generated higher revenue overall. Running a primary care office had become more expensive than when Richard Rutland did it, and family doctors could make most of their income by staying in their offices and seeing thirty or forty patients a day. In addition, the number of patients needing to be seen in the office was going up substantially as people now had insurance that allowed them to access primary care at low cost to themselves. Insurance companies placed pressure on family doctors to remain in the office all day, seeing their patients on a treadmill of one in-person visit after another, by turning the work of primary care into piece work—smaller pots of reimbursement given for each visit held, rather than what went on during the visit. This created perverse financial incentives for family doctors to eschew long, relationship-building visits with their patients in favor of fast-food-style primary care service delivery.

The downside for scope of work was that by no longer caring for patients when they showed up at the emergency room, family doctors lost access to specialists based in the hospital from whom they could learn more complex medicine. They also had to deal with the undermining of trust which resulted from patients no longer seeing their primary care doctors at a time when they were scared, vulnerable, and needing emergency treatment. Thus, patients lost confidence that some of their family doctors could do complex work.

Fast forward to the late 1990s when the specialty of hospital medicine—physicians who practice full-time, inpatient "primary care" (i.e., hospitalists)—came into existence, further taking away some of the remaining complex work of family doctors. There are now over 50,000 practicing hospitalists in the United States (Wachter and Goldman 2016). This growing army of inpatient doctors care for most of the family doctor's existing patients when those patients end up in the hospital. Part of what drove many family doctors away from hospital care as a normal part of their everyday practice was the economics of reimbursement. Similar to emergency medicine visits, a family physician's ability to generate revenue from multiple outpatient office visits outstrips what they could earn in the same time visiting one or two of their patients in the hospital on a given day (Hoff 2010). Like the case of losing emergency department exposure, no longer going to the hospital has negative effects on family doctors practicing in the community. It limits their potential to gain new clinical knowledge from specialists and strengthen the bonds between them and their patients.

There are other reasons for the narrowing of family doctor work. For instance, the efforts of gynecologists to become the "primary care" doctors for their pregnant patients, and the rising malpractice risks associated with family doctors doing fewer cases of obstetric care, have demotivated many family doctors from engaging in this work over time (Tong et al. 2013). Add to this the timing and time-commitment uncertainties of obstetrics—a labor and delivery can happen at any time, day or night, and can last for hours—and it's easy to see why family doctors who are working full-time to see patients in their offices have trouble absorbing the potential disruptions to their workdays that obstetrics poses.

The decline in obstetrical work for family doctors also illuminates another causal factor for the narrowing scope of practice—the shifting values and preferences for many working in the specialty. Younger physicians generally now value lifestyle and work-life balance to a greater extent than their predecessors. These shifting values are also shared by those becoming family doctors as well (Hoff 2010; Rege 2017). Younger doctors express a desire to work fewer hours; are more reluctant to take work home with them or be on regular call for patients during nights or weekends; and view medicine as a good 9-to-5 job rather than a 24-hour, 7-day-a-week calling (Dorsey et al. 2003; Shanafelt et al. 2015). The job and career-related preferences that derive from these values and beliefs do not align well with some portions of family practice work, such as obstetrics or emergency medicine that have high degrees of uncertainty as to when the work occurs. They also do not align with the ideal role of the family doctor that emphasizes being available to patients on nights and weekends, or the care manager role that requires family doctors to engage in administrative work on behalf of their patients.

Finally, there is the corporatization of family medicine work, seen mainly in the number of family doctors now working as salaried employees for larger organizations. Less than half of physicians now own their own practices, with younger physicians owning an even smaller percentage, and all physicians are becoming employees of larger groups in higher percentages over time (Kane 2019). Given the resource requirements to own a practice, most doctors are unwilling or unable to take the plunge. Most newly minted physicians become salaried employees because they carry large educational debt loads, have a desire for work-life balance, or are unable to gain access to enough viable independent practices in which they can buy into. A third of all US physicians now work as salaried employees of hospitals (Kane 2019). One recent American Medical Association survey reveals that almost 60 percent of all family doctors are working as salaried employees (Mazzolini 2019).

While becoming salaried employees of larger health care organizations may aid family doctors in their desire to work fewer hours, have good work-life balance, and avoid the hassles of owning a business, it can undermine their feeling of autonomy and their ability to engage in a wider scope of practice, should they so wish. This may not be a problem for some family doctors, as we will see. But for others, it becomes a growing source of dissatisfaction and burnout. It may reshape their professional identities in ways that are bad for their own sense of worth and the good of advancing their specialty. Working for hospitals and large health systems with specialty care at their nexus tends to deemphasize the importance of family doctors and the role of the comprehensive physician. The organization becomes the main contact for patients and seeks to develop a "relationship" with them that competes with the doctor (see Hoff 2017). It turns many primary care doctors into "loss leaders" for these organizations, that is, parts of the organization that earn less profit directly, but which help to feed patients into other parts of the specialty-based system where reimbursements and margins are higher. In this way, the family doctor's relationship with their patient becomes monetized, representing a valuable resource for larger health systems to acquire. Indeed, it is this motivation that has driven the rapid acquisition of physician practices by hospitals over the past decade (LaPointe 2019).

Low reimbursements for primary care, leading to lower family doctor compensation; big ideas like the Resource-Based Relative Value Scale, managed care, and the patient-centered medical home that were coopted by other interests and did not raise pay or status for family doctors; a primary care transformation led by Amazon thinking and dumbed-down primary care that creates cheaper, more accessible competition for family doctors and their practices; and a narrowing scope of work that undercuts their ideal of the comprehensive physician: these are the key contextual realities that have undermined family medicine's ability to thrive. There have been other realities, many related to the ones presented in this chapter—such as fewer US medical students choosing family medicine over the past twenty years, the continued public preoccupation with specialists and procedural medicine, and the explosion in medical knowledge—that make being a comprehensive family doctor so challenging.

Despite this adverse context, the specialty of family medicine has produced tens of thousands of dedicated doctors since the early 1970s—doctors who have lived up to the hype of the comprehensive physician, true to the ideal that those such as Richard Rutland fulfilled; and doctors who have begun their careers seeking to fulfill or at the least chase this ideal meaningfully. But as we will also see, there are many others who are less dogmatic and dogged who become family doctors. What motivates these individuals to become doctors? Why do they choose family medicine? By understanding better how this brand of doctor first comes into being, and the potential diversity involved in those who choose that brand, are there things we can learn about where family medicine is and where it may be headed? We turn to these questions next.

6/27/1997

Dr. Rutland,

...In 1975, my father was taken to the emergency room of the Fayette Hospital suffering from chest pains. You said it was one of the worst heart attacks you had ever seen and after a day or two had passed, he was not improving. Again, thanks to your dedication and perseverance, you "went the extra mile," called another doctor, got him on some new medication and he began to improve. As I remember it, you were there in the ICU most of the time until he started to get better. I call that saving his life. My respect and admiration for you as a person and a physician goes beyond measure. Thank you for helping me to have my daddy still with me after more than 20 years have passed....

In loving gratitude,

Sarah S.

Patient letter to Dr. Rutland upon his retirement, 1997 (Rutland Papers, Center for the History of Family Medicine [CHFM])

THREE

Altruists and Accidental Doctors

Why They Become (Family) Doctors

IT IS NOT SURPRISING that young people might enter medical school and choose family medicine out of a general desire to do something good and to help people in meaningful ways. I found those motivations in some of the family doctors I interviewed. However, I was surprised at how small a number of doctors it ended up being. Only about a quarter of those with whom I spoke expressed this desire, some younger and some older. A second surprise was that even for those expressing an altruistic motivation, most also stated that they did not experience a burning passion or drive to become a physician or a family physician in order to fulfill it. It just happened to be a career choice that generally aligned with helping people in their young 20-year-old minds, and it did not always present itself as an option right away. They did not stumble blindly into it. But they also did not dream of it incessantly.

Adam is a family doctor in his mid-thirties who fancies himself as a Richard Rutland–style country doctor. He comes across as a levelheaded guy, a straight shooter who is serious about his views and what he does. He practices in a small town in western New York as an employee of a larger health care system. He does his work in a rural setting where he also lives with his own family, a wife and two kids under the age of 5, and he's been in the same town since finishing his residency. As a family doctor, he is in the thick of it, a community-based medical practice. Adam tries to practice generalist or comprehensive family medicine in his practice, which means he seeks to take care of all of his patients' needs, including mental health care, chronic disease management, preventive care, and many forms of acute care. He has patients of all ages in his practice. While he does not deliver babies or do procedures, he does engage in special work like concussion management with young local athletes. He is aware that burnout and working too much is the cause of the dissatisfaction many doctors feel, but he is satisfied in his job, in part, because of the well-rounded work he performs every day.

He recalls that he first thought of being a doctor as a young child. But it was the same way many children may think of being a doctor or firefighter or professional athlete. Not understanding what it really means or how hard it is to accomplish. He did not think much more about it until he was older and found that he had an abstract interest to do something to better peoples' lives.

> I was always interested in being a doctor, at least I can remember back to sixth grade saying that I was interested in going into medicine and being a doctor. I think it was because I liked science and I also liked people, pretty standard things. I enjoyed those things, and I found in high school and in college I still enjoyed those things. In college, going through some of the more difficult prerequisites, there were obviously times when you wondered, is this really what I wanna do? (Adam, early-career family doctor)

Adam mentions that this idea of liking people and wanting to help them in some way has stayed with him through his whole life. It led him initially to consider entering the clergy, not becoming a physician.

> I also was a religion major and I considered going into ministry. . . . I think that medicine and ministry are both fields of—they tend to be people who care deeply about people. They tend to be people who enjoy learning. They tend to be idealistic people, especially at the start. They tend to be people who have a strong idea about right and wrong, about ethics, and about using their skills to care for people and provide good,

and they tend to be fields where there is a sense of the gravity of the field. In some respect you feel like this is an important thing, life and death or a significant impact that you're providing. (Adam)

Young and old alike, the altruists share the same attribute, namely, that they ultimately chose a medical and family medicine career because it aligned well with their humanistic and charitable motivations. At the same time, they did not convey a sense to me that medicine was the only way to satisfy these specific motivations. Adam and a couple of others in the group I spoke with might have become priests. Others would have considered becoming public health workers, nurses, social workers, or international aid workers if they had not chosen medicine. For them, a medical career did not start out as the end all be all. It did not even start out as the first serious career choice most of them thought of to fulfill their motivation to do good.

I had an advisor who was a similar faith to me, same denomination and everything, and his advice to me at the time, as he got to know me and I was in one of his classes, he said, "You would be a good seminary student. You would probably be a good minister. Be a doctor. We need doctors and lawyers and mailmen."

That was starting the process, that people that I looked up to still sort of thought that [medicine] was the career that would be valuable, and I never did feel a true call to ordained ministry, to be a minister. So, then as things progressed and fell into line, I was still most interested in going into medical school. (Adam)

Adam was leaning toward being a family doctor when he went to medical school. His experiences seeing the different brands of doctor while he was there made up his mind.

I would say that I'd always been kind of interested in more the primary care thing, and I figured out I did not want to be a surgeon. I did not enjoy standing for long periods of time staring into small holes. So, I kind of had known my mentality and approach was gonna be more for some sort of primary care. I went into clerkships thinking if I liked internal, I'll do that. If I like kids, I'll do peds [pediatrics]. If I like psych,

I'll do psych. If I like the ER, I can do that. And if I like everything then I'll probably do family medicine, and I did find that I enjoyed the breadth and depth, so that's why I went into family medicine. (Adam)

As we spoke, he continued to focus on the human side of being a doctor, and how family medicine fulfilled that human aspect of the profession the most.

At least for me, in family medicine it's very much helping folks to cope with the day-to-day. There's a strong aspect of feeling like you're trying to heal someone, you're trying to help them in that respect, and I think that's very much the role of a pastor in many cases. For me, my grandfather was a minister. My wife's mother is a retired minister, and my mother went back to seminary when I was in medical school, so we have pretty strong ties to religious communities. (Adam)

He entered a rural medicine training program for family doctors during residency, which helped fuel his interest in doing real family medicine within a small community, like a Richard Rutland. Having grown up in a small town, this aligned well with his own identity.

I graduated from college in 2004. I had taken my MCAT fairly late. I took the later session and my applications were a little late, so I got into SUNY Upstate on the waitlist in 2004, so I started school there and, yeah, so I went to Upstate, I did well there, liked it. I come from a very small town, my high school graduated forty-four students, and so I came—and I'd always kinda said I was probably interested in practicing in a rural area. And so, I joined that program. In third and fourth year I did the traditional program. I spent nine months living in a small town in upstate New York and working with a physician at the hospital there. I did my family medicine, my general surgery, orthopedics, ENT, all of those things I did at the community hospital there. So, that certainly formed sort of my thinking—and I had a pretty good idea by that time that I wanted to go into primary care. (Adam)

The Promise and Peril of Pursuing an Altruistic Career Outlet

There were several more like Adam who I interviewed—small town kids whose experiences in tight-knit communities growing up made them conscious of having a career that could allow them to give back in some way. Others did not come from small towns but still felt altruistic. For example, Renee is a third-year family medicine resident working in Boston. She is 30 years old, a few years older than the typical third-year resident. She comes across during the interview as mature and serious about her chosen path. Unlike Adam, she is an *urban* altruist, committed to working in the inner city and caring for disadvantaged populations, poorer and often Black and Latino. She grew up in Boston, in a well-to-do home, with a mom who was a lawyer and social justice advocate and a dad who was a doctor. She has a new husband and 5-week-old baby. She is taking some time off before starting her first full-time job at a Boston-area primary care practice. Her residency is with a safety net provider who engages in the difficult care delivery work that defines big city existence— working with the poor and underserved, often people in poorer health and living conditions. She mentions wanting to be a doctor early in life. But medical school was never a foregone conclusion for her.

> Okay, so my dad is a physician. He's in geriatrics and palliative care, and so when I was very young I wanted to be a doctor and then I kind of had that STEM sort of fall-out thing that happens to girls in the seventh and ninth grade, and I decided I did not like science at all, whatsoever, because I wasn't good at it. So I did not want to do that [become a doctor]. I actually moved in high school and there was a problem with my transcript, and I didn't end up taking any science classes after tenth grade, and nobody ever caught on and I thought it was great.
>
> In undergrad I studied international relations and American studies; and I was thinking about doing some non-profit management which is more in line with what my mom did. She was a human rights lawyer and then did the non-profit work later. I took what is essentially like Rocks for Jocks kind of classes to fulfill my science requirements in college; zoology was my real one science class. I landed an internship [after

college] in Ecuador doing observational health research, which I thought was exactly what I wanted to do with my life and did resource planning with plantation workers. . . . I hated it. I spent two months doing that and I had one very close friend who was a medical resident, and I kept thinking, like wow, look at her; she does these tangible, incredible things that make a difference, and she can see the results straight away. I'm doing this work that takes ten or twenty years [to see a difference]. (Renee, third-year family medicine resident)

She had a privileged upbringing and experiences some degree of guilt because of that, one might say, which feeds into her altruistic mentality. Unprovoked during the interview, she talks about how at one point after college she tried to sort that out a bit for herself.

I went to a bunch of regional social justice trainings. . . . [I] thought about my privilege and my guilt, and I went through a lot of stages of guilt about it, and now it's not so much guilt. I think, yes, having privilege does make me feel like I want to work for those who don't but so does the rest of my upbringing where my mom was just a fierce advocate and you know she didn't have these kinds of things growing up. She ate hot dog buns with ketchup for dinner, for like the entire time she was in college. (Renee)

Renee tells me at the end of our conversation that she is not sure how her family medicine career will move forward, in part because her altruistic interests are not all that fully clear, even to her. Others with whom I spoke, particularly the younger doctors, came across the same way. When asked to think more deeply on how they specifically would use medicine and then family medicine to serve some socially beneficial purpose, most were vague in their responses, that is, they liked public health work, they wanted a job where they could feel like they were helping people directly, they wanted a career with a mission, and they wanted to be in a powerful position to advocate for others.

I took the MCAT before I went off to the Peace Corps. . . . I wasn't in any medical field in the Peace Corps. I was teaching high school. . . . I kind of figured it out there that I wanted to go back to medical school, that I at least wanted to go back to school in some capacity, and that I really enjoyed one-on-one interactions with people and one-on-one level service. And so those two things kind of came together to mean medicine. It was, yeah, I guess a sense of service, a sense of good luck and privilege and a chance to use that one way or another, and a way to use that meaningfully in a way that would be fulfilling. (Sean, early-career family doctor)

I started in undergraduate, my goal was actually to be an environmental biologist, and do something about the ecosystem, and all that. Then I went on a trip to Uganda, in the middle of college, with a volunteer mission group. It was in the height of HIV in Uganda, at its worst. This is in the mid-90s. And at that point, I just felt like I wanted to do something to help people in a more direct way. And so, medicine became a little more appealing, and I decided to go to med school right after that. (Scott, mid-career family doctor)

Some of the altruists give me pause. Their motivations for becoming doctors and family doctors are noble. They seem like the kind of people we all wish would become doctors. Yet I wonder about their ability to avoid outcomes like burnout and job dissatisfaction as they attempt to work in ways that fulfill their goal of helping people who need it and being there for them. In a delivery system that will take as much as it can from a doctor, family doctors particularly, and not think twice about it, I wonder if their vague sense of wanting to help people can stand up to crushing workloads, reduced autonomy, and a health care system often designed to get in the way of helping people. I wonder if they can keep their head in the game when the career does not turn out the way they think—when they start to realize that the true family medicine role is often all-consuming, especially when caring for disadvantaged populations.

One altruist raised these questions for me, because he has been through the proverbial fire. Luke, a mid-career family doctor and altruist, has treated underserved populations throughout his career. He has traveled extensively to other countries practicing his medicine and has worked in New York City community health centers for years doing fuller-scope family medicine for disadvantaged patients. Working in a community health center, in a big city no less, is no easy job for a doctor; it's one of the toughest places around to ply the family medicine trade.

He has worked for Doctors Without Borders and for the Indian Health Service. He has put in his time living the family medicine ideal of trying to serve a larger community purpose. He deserves a lot of credit. He has logged many work hours over his career doing difficult things, and he probably has not gotten paid near to what he should have relative to his specialist colleagues. People think all doctors are highly paid, perhaps, but try doing their work day in and day out and you might realize the pay makes up for only part of all that mental and physical effort.

Luke seems like a good guy, another straight shooter, honest as the day is long. We talk on a cold January day at a family medicine conference in upstate New York, off in the corner of the hotel where the conference is being held. He comes across as relaxed. Still, there is an intensity laying under that calm demeanor. He tells me during our interview with a quiet fervency that he burned out pretty good recently from his community health center job. He has thought about his situation. His brutal honesty about it gives me pause. I do not often hear physicians talk so plainly about their own condition.

> I was walking to work [in New York City] and I wasn't gonna jump in front of the truck. But if the truck hit me and I didn't have to go to work that day, it would be okay. That was one day. And then that kinda happened for several days in a row. . . . And it felt like there was no room in my life for me. Every day I would wake up and be like, "How am I gonna get through this day?" I was doing sometimes forty-hour days, from when the woman came in until when she delivered. Sometimes I'd be in the clinic from eight in the morning until ten at night. Then it turned into this kind of passive suicidality.
>
> I went to my boss and I'm like, "I need to take some time." I had all this vacation time built up. I was just working like crazy. I was the only person doing deliveries in my program and I was the director of obstetrics. And we're only supposed to take two weeks at a time and I sort of pled my case. "I need three weeks. I need four weeks." I didn't give all the details.
>
> I went to Sri Lanka by myself. I just hung out in these Buddhist temples. I purposefully went by myself. Other people were like, "I'll go with you." I'm like, "No, I need to go alone." I just needed to meditate.

Towards the end of the trip I was on this empty beach. There were a few fishermen down at the end of it. And I was wading in the Indian Ocean and I had this moment of clarity: "I want more of this and less of that. I'm gonna go home and quit my job."

I actually told my boss [of a New York community health center] I was quitting. I was gonna take a year off and just do yoga and meditate and not do anything medical and just kind of try to save myself. But this job from New Zealand fell in my lap and it was perfect because it was four days a week. It was 9:00 to 5:00. It let me be in a beautiful place for nine months where I could sorta do all that kind of self-reflection stuff. Minimal call. (Luke, mid-career family doctor)

Luke is now a full-blooded career pragmatist in survival mode. He fends for himself first with his choices, and the interests of his underserved patients and the larger family medicine specialty second. Given how poorly he felt at one time, he does not feel this is a bad thing. Take care of yourself first, or you cannot take care of anyone else, he opines to me during our discussion. Hard to argue with that logic. He is still an altruist, but from our chat, I get a strong whiff of uncertainty toward how he sees the future for himself as a family doctor. There is some ambivalence that bleeds through his words. Some detachment from family medicine work that perhaps was not there before he burned out.

Do the altruists set themselves up for greater disappointment with the family medicine career? Especially given the nobler but ill-defined expectations they have about what that career can provide them, and a somewhat more naïve way of thinking about it to start? Richard Rutland probably thought like an altruist at an early age and saw medicine in this way. But Richard Rutland came of age as a family doctor when the health care system, though not fully kind to generalists, still allowed them greater autonomy over their practice and finances. It supported them in engaging in work that was more holistic for patients, fuller in scope, and richly rewarding. It was not the health care system of 2021. Rutland's system allowed family doctors to cultivate long-term relationships with their patients and reap the benefits of those relationships. It gave them prestige in their communities. It compensated them well enough. Rutland also did not have hundreds of thousands of dollars of debt to pay back. He did not have reams of paperwork to complete each day. He was more in control of how he did his job.

He also was not a millennial child reared in a complex society where the rewards of too much hard work and sacrificing for one's career are increasingly questioned, and do not seem to many to make up for what they take from people. The altruists who went into medicine and family medicine from the 1970s onward have seen less of Rutland's type of health care system over time. Yet, they have been asked to sacrifice more personally for the chance to be a family doctor. Then again, maybe Rutland also had a different mindset about his calling, and for whatever reason was more willing to do what it took to be that altruistic kind of doctor, compared to the doctors of today. Maybe he was willing to make the sacrifices necessary without asking for something for himself in return. That is one mystery we are dealing with here when we compare family doctors like him to today's breed.

The Accidental (Family) Doctors Who Seek a Good Career Option

There were a group of approximately thirty interviewees that I came to know as "accidental doctors." These doctors recalled nondescript motivations for going to medical school and choosing family medicine, such as (a) they should be doing something worthy and prestigious to justify their "book smarts," and (b) they wanted career flexibility and the ability to have options down the road. These were not strong motivations for choosing either medicine or family medicine, as they recalled them. Rather, they sounded like personal rationales for making such an expensive (on many levels for them) career choice. A few of the accidental doctors were also altruists. Most were not. Rather, they were people who felt that they fell into a medical career, and became family doctors by a mixture of chance, some small amount of premeditation, and being afforded a rarer opportunity because of their upbringing (e.g., doctors already in the family or no educational debt from undergraduate) and academic preparation.

For some of the self-described "science nerds" who were good with numbers and formulas, the prototypical career of having a PhD and working in a research lab, away from most human contact, was not what they wanted. Many knew that from the start. Others found out once they worked in labs during college or right after. They knew they were talented in science, but pursuing that talent as research scientists came to be less palatable. For others who had multiple doctors in their family and had been raised around doctors, there was the feeling that becoming a doctor was a safe yet honorable career choice, one where you got people's respect.

For a few there was a personal experience with the health system that helped push them along. Others carried little debt because their parents or scholarships had paid for undergraduate schooling, so they chose medicine in part because they had more financial freedom. Still others believed that medicine and family medicine would allow them, as they got older, to not be locked into one overly strict career path. This seemed ironic given the personal and financial sacrifices involved in becoming a doctor generally. Some would see medicine as a strict career path.

Brian and Billy are accidental doctors: third-year, twenty-something medical students in upstate New York who are good friends. They are smart kids and are easy to talk with. During my first few discussions with them, they both indicated an interest in becoming family doctors. They come from different backgrounds. Brian's parents are immigrants, and his father is a retired surgeon. His mom is a lawyer. Two of his siblings are already doctors and another is a dentist. A successful family by any definition—pedigree everywhere—and a lot of achievement that Brian has grown up around. Here is someone that will be compelled to think of a high prestige occupation whether he wants to or not. Because of his exposure to a physician household, Brian not surprisingly talks about the respect and security that comes with being a doctor.

> Basically, I think it was more of a social capital kind of thing. Doctors are very well respected by the general public, in general, you know? It's a safe career. If you have that MD, you have a pretty good chance of having an

income, and a good income at that. So those two things I think drove my choice. (Brian, third-year medical student)

On the other hand, Billy comes from a working-class background. His dad is a retired cop. His mom works as a cashier. He had a real blue-collar upbringing. I expect Billy to talk about the same motivation. After all, that should be part of the allure for a working-class kid like him—the respect and prestige of being a physician, the social mobility and all that. But he focuses instead on the way his academic involvement in science and a personal experience brought medicine as a career into view.

I guess probably when I was first in high school deciding what to go into for college. At first, I wanted to go into film actually. I didn't necessarily want to do anything science related. I liked science, but I didn't really see it as a career, necessarily. Then, at around the same time . . . my friend from high school ended up developing cancer. . . . And then, when I was looking at different majors in college, one of the things that peaked my interest for that reason was nuclear medicine because one of the things they were advertising was its [use] for imaging for cancer patients. So, that's when I selected that as my undergrad major not thinking about graduate school or anything necessarily at the time. I was also interested in psychology. I picked up that as a second major. Then, by the end of the year, I was thinking of being a psychiatrist as opposed to a nuclear medicine technologist. It wasn't really a direct path and a lot of it was kind of like roundabout. It wasn't as clear cut for me until a little bit later that that's actually something that I wanted to do. Nobody in my family was in health care at all. I didn't really talk to anybody personally about it. (Billy, third-year medical student)

Brian and Billy do not talk as if medicine was a slam-dunk career choice. Both initially wanted to work in the arts.

I was a theater major and a theology major double, and when I told that to my parents and started really thinking about it, it became pretty clear that it would be hard to make a career out of that. I started doing some research at a local cancer hospital and in the meantime, my father was diagnosed with gastric cancer. The combination of not having a real career path from two of my passions [theater and theology], and being pretty interested in cancer research and my father being diagnosed with cancer, kind of made me want to take the MCAT and apply. (Brian)

The science angle is also significant. Both tell me they were good in science, and perhaps this made going for medicine an easier choice and a better fit. After all, if you are not adept in biology, chemistry, and physics, which inform our understanding of all life, you are not going to grasp or succeed in medical training. You also probably will not like it very much. This explanation comes up a lot in my interviews with the accidental doctors in the group; their affinity for scientific fields seemed to limit their career options to less than a handful of viable and worthy jobs. But if you are good at science, and like science, you may feel the need to engage in a science-oriented career. It is that simple.

Paula is a second-year family medicine resident working in the Boston area. Like Billy and Brian, she also did not have some grand plan to be a doctor. She does not come across as some gung ho family doctor, at least not the kind willing to pursue Richard Rutland–type duties and work hours. But she possesses a combination of those features mentioned above that made a career as a physician logical. Her parents are both engineers, so there is pedigree here as well. Pedigree comes up a lot with the accidental doctors. They don't necessarily need to have doctors in the family, per se, but having family members in good occupations creates a family aura of success. She has no undergraduate debt, so there is financial freedom. She saw medicine as a somewhat flexible career where you could do different things. She was also a science nerd.

I guess I went straight through from college to medical school. I went to Cornell, and I was studying physics. I didn't have that much exposure to medicine in high school or even really in college, but . . . I think a lot of people in college who are good at school and ambitious think, "Maybe I should be a doctor." I don't think it was very informed, but it was on my list of things I might want to do. But then, I also thought maybe I was going to do research, so I was doing research in biomedical sciences with a physics focus, because I was interested in lasers.

I didn't really like how little interaction with people you get when doing research. I was working in a basement mostly on computers. I thought that maybe medicine would be more satisfying because you would be working with the people that you're trying to help, so you would get a little bit more immediate gratification. That's how I decided to go to medical school. Then, I went to Penn State, and I didn't really know what kind of medicine I wanted to do at that point. I met a couple people who were family medicine doctors early on in medical school, who also had done undergrad and, actually, PhDs in physics. They were like, "Oh, you did physics. We did physics. You should do family medicine." I just liked them, so I started thinking about maybe doing family medicine. (Paula, second-year family medicine resident)

She tells me during the interview that her parents did not push her into medicine. Her mom especially had reservations about her becoming a family doctor. Her mom thought she might want to choose a specialty where you could do more research. Or perhaps earn a bit more money commensurate with the investment in training. Very pragmatic stuff. Her father stayed out of the discussion. But she said she liked the family doctors she met in medical school, they seemed like good people to her. How much of seeing good people in various occupations influences all of us to do that same something with our lives? Probably more than we think. She had no medical school debt either because her parents also paid for medical school.

I didn't have any debt. I mean, I think it definitely made me feel free to choose whatever I wanted to do without having to worry about what the different incomes were, because if you have no debt, all of it is great. Some of my friends in medical school who were trying to decide . . . we would do the calculation together [of the debt payback over time] and it was like, "Oh, wow." Especially one of my friends who's married . . . he needs to support his whole family. (Paula)

Paula likes the flexibility of family medicine work, at least as she sees it. She does not want to do only traditional outpatient, one-on-one patient care. She is potentially interested in getting involved in population health work and working more with groups of patients on multidisciplinary health care teams. She is willing to have jobs where she is not the boss, or even the lead clinician. She thinks the family medicine career can offer some of that work variety.

Hedging Bets and Flexing the Family Medicine Career

A lot of others who I interview, particularly those at earlier stages in their careers, talk about the flexibility advantage of family medicine. *Flexibility*—now there is an interestingly used word among these doctors. It seems like the flexibility many end up talking about, particularly the younger family doctors, is not the flexibility of being a comprehensive physician in the mold of the traditional family doctor archetype, or the sort of flexibility the specialty would like to hear its members embrace—doing lots of different kinds of clinical work, for example, but in the context of well-defined and stable patient relationships.

Instead, it is a flexibility defined as being able to choose different types of jobs and clinical settings in which to work, for example, outpatient family medicine in a traditional physician-centric practice; urgent care centers; hospital medicine; perhaps even an administrative position. It's the flexibility to work part-time in several jobs and offices rather than one, or to do shift work as opposed to an everyday nine-to-five schedule. The flexibility to call your own shots in terms of when to work, where to work, and how to work. The flexibility to earn higher salaries doing multiple part-time jobs simultaneously, or to be able to move from one job to another higher paying one at their leisure.

Bianca is one such younger family doctor who likes the specialty for this kind of flexibility. She is in her mid-thirties and has been practicing for about five years. She lives and works in New York. Another who comes from a successful family, one of her sisters is a doctor and another is a chemical engineer, Bianca went to medical school in the Caribbean and owes almost $400,000 in student loans. She sounds pragmatic about her motivation to be a doctor and a family doctor.

Coming out of [family medicine] residency, I had always planned to do part-time primary care, and part-time urgent care. . . . And I told myself, well, initially, I'll take the walk into just urgent care alone because the schedule will be a lot easier, and I'll probably be able to do full-time hours with fewer days a week, and have more time off. And that's what I did, I signed on for a full-time urgent care job, and within a year I signed on to do part-time primary care, and then I was doing the part-time primary care two days a week, and three days a week of the urgent care.

I gave myself some time off, and after two years in the urgent care center that I was working at, they asked me to come on as their medical director for their two sites. The bump in pay, and the step up on the ladder—I really wanted to take it, and so I asked the primary care place that I was working at if I could take a step back and do one day a week, and they countered with how about you work for us full-time instead. Because [they said] one day a week is not what we're looking for, and we really want you to come on, [but] I was really kind of interested in seeing where this medical director role would take me, and so that's what I've been doing full-time for the last year and a half-ish. I'm really enjoying it. I do miss the primary care aspect of family medicine. I intend to go back to it at some point, but early in my career, a medical director opportunity was not something that I could pass up. (Bianca, early-career family doctor)

She owes a lot of money, like a number of the younger doctors I interviewed. Hundreds of thousands of dollars that takes years to pay back. A house mortgage before you have a house. This kind of career flexibility was important to making her family medicine choice. She does not want to work full-time for a traditional office-based practice where her hours will be longer and workload higher. Many older family doctors, particularly ones that have worked in this more traditional primary care practice setting their whole careers, probably would look at someone like Bianca and not recognize or applaud her brand of flexibility in her family medicine career. For them the definition of flexibility is not about a different type of job or employment setting, doing primary care work that perhaps is more schedule-friendly and less intense, or working several different part-time jobs at once.

Instead, it is the kind of flexibility described above that is centered on everyday work variety, that is, the different types of clinical work, simple and complex, time consuming and not, in which you can engage with a given group of patients that you have known for a long time. It's the kind of flexibility in which Richard Rutland engaged as a comprehensive family doctor, doing lots of different things, and working for his patients and the community in which he worked and lived. Another person I interviewed, Vic, thought of flexibility in this more old-fashioned way when he became a family doctor in the 1970s. He is almost 70 now and still practices full-time. He has always done traditional outpatient work in a private practice, and he has taught younger family doctors for decades. He is one of the altruists who became a physician by relative accident.

I'm one of five boys in the family. We lived on the south shore of Long Island. I was born in Brooklyn, and my dad moved our family out. I was born in 1950. My original career choice was the clergy. I spent four years of . . . high school at a minor preparatory seminary in my local diocese. The school that I went to no longer exists because it was closed, but I got a good education, and I thought I might have had a vocation to that sort of work. But I decided, as I was finishing up my high school years, that, for a couple of reasons, not the least of which was I wanted to do something that would be less tied to a particular religion, a little more secular, but still had a sense of mission, [I would not join the clergy]. When I looked around, medicine seemed to fit that bill. I had nobody in my family who had ever been in medicine or nursing.

I was originally going to be an English major [in college] coming out of the seminary, but then I changed, and they accepted me as a pre-med. And my first year I did okay. I lived off campus, and I commuted. My second year, at Fordham University, I lived on campus and I struggled a little bit with some of the pre-med math courses. For a while, I thought that I would change from being pre-med and go into something more in languages or liberal arts. I did that for a semester and then eventually changed back to pre-med.

I picked family medicine for the same reason I still like practicing it today. It has variety. It allows me to maintain an overall competency in a number of fields, although as I've grown older in family medicine, I've recognized that [there are] some areas in that big, broad discipline that I'm going to do better [in] than others. When I was first going through training, I liked the fact that family medicine was one of the few disciplines that maintained the structure, at least in the first year, that was very much like the old rotating [general practice] internship. You did four months of medicine. You did a couple of months of surgery, a couple of months of OB, a couple of months of peds. You were in the emergency department. You got a good grounding quickly in all the traditional disciplines that comprised general practice. I never thought that my work as a family doc would make me an expert in everything; it couldn't because medicine was far more complex—even back when I started, as opposed to now, where it's incredibly complex. But I wanted to be able [to] address a lot of the concerns of the patients, and I also wanted to know how to make a good referral, and I thought family medicine was a good fit. I worried that in other disciplines I might get bored just seeing the same thing. (Vic, late-career family doctor)

Unlike Vic, who was an accidental doctor that went all in on trying to create a traditional comprehensive family doctor career, I have come to think of Bianca and some accidental doctors like her, the younger ones especially, as "bet-hedgers." The bet-hedgers choose medicine and family medicine because they have an innate desire as young people to give themselves future options. Options in terms of how they want to enact their careers, the kinds of jobs they may wish to have, the need for work-life balance, the desire to have the security of a good income, and the ability to have multiple career paths if they so choose. Among doctors under 35, this bet-hedging motivation was talked about in the interviews as much as was the motivation of being an altruist.

Bet-hedging reflects the idea of engaging in a safer, more sustainable career that can be manipulated to meet the expectations of the individual. It's not the normative expectations of the larger specialty or medical profession. It is odd to think of medicine as a "safe" career, given what is involved in becoming a doctor. The sacrifices, financial and otherwise, that are involved. But for these chosen few, this is how they see it. It's not a calling that comes from the drive to be altruistic or make a profound difference in society, but a career path that gives them a decent, well-paying job for life. A safe path where they can still do interesting work.

What they really want is what the management literature calls a "sustainable career" (De Vos et al. 2018; De Vos 2015). Such a career idea focuses on people acting in highly pragmatic, self-interested ways in their job and work decisions, mainly to feel enhanced personal control in larger career environments that feel uncertain (Lawrence et al. 2015). Two concepts in this theory are worth considering when thinking about our family doctors. First is the concept of employability, which means that people want a strong guarantee of future employment over the course of their entire work lives (Lawrence et al. 2015). The second concept of workability refers to how "viable" a career is over the course of one's lifetime, based subjectively on that person's expectations of what they desire from it. Viability means a lot of things, like the ability to have job satisfaction, avoid burnout, achieve work-life balance, and have work that is appropriately interesting and autonomous. It is clear for many of the younger doctors that the choice of family medicine is especially driven, in part, by the idea that such a medical specialty is perhaps more sustainable than other ones.

The accidental doctors and their smaller subset of bet-hedgers are pertinent to this story about family medicine. Why? Because their motivations for becoming doctors and family doctors, and their career thinking, do not align ideally with a medical specialty who still defines the working role of its members rigidly and one dimensionally. This does not mean that accidental doctors—the old, the young, the (mostly younger) bet-hedgers—do not ultimately commit to that rigid role definition, one the Richard Rutlands of the world might favor. As we will see, many do. Yet even some of those who enact their roles as "true believers" at one point in time, and try to fulfill the comprehensive physician ideal, turn to more sustainable career decision making as time goes on, as we shall see. As more family doctors embrace the sustainable career pursuit, further balkanization of the specialty occurs.

When I catch up with good friends and medical students Billy and Brian several months later by phone, suddenly their career choices have diverged. Both told me earlier they were interested in choosing family medicine as their specialty, and for similar reasons. But Brian is becoming a pediatrician now, in part because his early experience working alongside family doctors convinced him that the job is too difficult to do the way he would like to. And he's worried it may make him unhappy; in his mind, it's a lot of paperwork and adult patients who, no matter how much you commit to them as a doctor, will not change their unhealthy lifestyles or listen to your advice or guidance. He thinks dealing with kids will be more rewarding and probably easier, and he believes he can make a bigger difference. So Brian is thinking about his career in a sustainable way even before picking family medicine.

Billy still wants to be a family doctor. He sees the same challenges with adult patients that Brian does, but he thinks it is the kind of work role that will give him personal fulfillment. At least right now, he is fine with that traditional, full-scope role and all that it brings with it, good and bad. He also has seen something in his family medicine work that he likes a lot.

> I think for me it was just, I want to actually do more stuff with family medicine. It [my family medicine rotation] kind of confirmed what I already had a decent idea about. Having the same patients for a while. I saw that when I was on my family med clerkship; the same attendings are taking care of their patients in the hospital, and it's just such a different, new, interesting environment—to be able to see the patient's face light up when they see that . . . an attending that they're used to seeing for the past . . . ten or twenty years, or even more than that, is the one taking care of them . . . when they're really sick. That they already have that trusting relationship built—they already have established rapport with that person. Like they walk into the room and they're starting to talk about their kids. Like it's a definitely a different environment than some of the other rotations I've been on. (Billy)

Of course, it is the Billys of family medicine that the specialty and its visionaries have always hoped to turn out in greater numbers, in order to maintain the specialty's preferred identity and fulfill its counterculture goals and aspirations. An army of young Billys willing to plant a stake in the ground, do full-service outpatient and inpatient medicine, make their community a better place, and excel at relational care delivery. Replacing those ahead of them who have done the same, like Vic. Making medicine more humane and personal for patients.

Goals, visions, and aspirations are all one thing—wonderful sounding phrases and narratives built to inspire and motivate. But for the fledgling specialty of family medicine in those early years of the late 1960s and early 1970s, fighting an uphill battle against the rest of the medical profession for its rightful place in our health care system, words were not enough. To gain a foothold in the profession, acquire needed resources, attract young medical students, and assure public support, the specialty made a number of strategic choices and promises to those it was hoping to sell on its ideal. At the same time such choices and promises were fueling the early rise of family medicine, they were also sowing the seeds of later stagnation: the specialty's decreased attractiveness to newer generations of medical students and its ambivalent reputation with the public.

It is this general dilemma of unfulfilled potential that will be dealt with a little later. But first, we must understand this short-sighted strategic behavior in greater detail. What drove it and why, and within what context did it occur?

Dr. R.O. Rutland, Jr.,

I'll never forget the time, over 10 years ago. My daughter and her baby, from Lake Charles were visiting me. The baby developed a high fever in the late afternoon, we called you and by the time we could get to Fayette, your office was closed, but you checked the baby anyway. Told us what to do for her, and to report back the next morning on her condition. I was so relieved.

Then in October of '94 my husband was in the Fayette Hospital a week before he died. He was not one of your patients. However, you came into his room three different nights and sat and talked with me five or ten minutes, even though you were not his doctor. I'll never forget you being so thoughtful, kind, and caring.

Kathleen S.

Patient letter to Dr. Rutland upon his retirement, 1997 (Rutland Papers, Center for the History of Family Medicine [CHFM])

FOUR

Saying Goodbye to the General Doctor

IT BEGAN AS A GRAND and noble idea. But it would succumb to the same mistakes other occupations, especially those with strong advocates, make. Too much promise making, unrealistic expectations, shortsighted decisions, and ideological grandstanding. Yet it was also brazen and timely, and it possessed the unbridled hope that motivates people to do new things. Make no mistake, the idea of a family medicine specialty was opportune. America in the 1960s was in upheaval. A window had opened for new, radical ideas about social justice, equality, and the lifting of everyone's boat for the collective goal of a better life for all Americans (Starr 1982). As Gayle Stephens, one of family practice's intellectual founders, noted years later about the late 1960s:

> What I remember most clearly . . . was my sense of excitement and optimism about changes in medical care; it seemed the nation was prepared to reform its chronic problems—the doctor shortage, escalating costs, unjust distribution of medical services to rural and inner-city populations, and fragmentation of care among generalists and specialists. Our Sedgwick County Medical Society had led a successful campaign in 1962 to 1963 to immunize free of charge all willing citizens with the oral polio vaccine.

The Medicare and Medicaid amendments had been passed by Congress in 1965, and the "Summer of Love" was happening in San Francisco. . . . The catalyst for Family Practice, in my view, was the reform ethos of the 1960s that tapped into deep springs of American idealism and values—agrarianism, humanism, civil rights, feminism, and distributive justice. These ideals and values shaped the new discipline in ways not imagined by organized medicine. The new programs attracted faculty and medical students because they had a new vision of medical education and the roles of physicians and other health care professionals. (Stephens 2010, pp. S5–S7)

Stephens, like other early family medicine champions, was a visionary. But he also saw the writing on the wall. The push to a family medicine specialty, one that could be accorded equal status with other clinical specialties, was not only borne out of a lofty ideological desire to establish a more robust, better-trained generalist. Strategically, it was likely a last-gasp attempt to ensure the survival of that type of physician in the United States, regardless of what they were called. This was not something shouted from the mountain tops by people like Stephens or other headstrong leaders of the family medicine movement, in part because they sought to distance the new specialty from the traditional general practitioner's increasingly negative connotation. They wanted to support a new type of generalist doctor without supporting the older kind.

The new family doctor was going to be a generalist, albeit a better-trained, more narrowly construed one. The definitions that would end up being put forth for the new specialty, and the reality of who owned other clinical turf, dictated that outcome. But from the outset, family physicians were pitched as comprehensive doctors. Doctors who could care for patients holistically and manage all their health care needs. In this sense, the push to dispense with the general practitioner and replace them with the family practitioner was a bold, calculated, but also desperate move. An attempt to sell patients, policy makers, and the rest of medicine on the recreation of a medical species on the verge of extinction. In large part because that species had been left behind in the intellectual, technical, and procedural advances of modern medicine. It was a species now looked down upon by many, even a good portion of those doing it. For family medicine's early advocates and founders, the main strategic thrust was to embark on a serious rebranding exercise for those who would do primary care medicine. It would be reinvention at its finest.

Nero Fiddles while Rome Burns: The Rapid Decline of General Practice in America

Much of the field of general practice had fooled itself between 1945 and 1965 into thinking it was a going concern long term, claiming to have some support for this view. There was the argument that general practitioners (GPs) did indeed perform a lot of complex medical work and had a wide scope of practice. In defense of that argument, a 1948 American Academy of General Practice (AAGP) survey of select members showed 86 percent of respondents handling obstetrics cases, with the average number of babies delivered annually by a given GP being fifty-one (American Academy of General Practice 1948b). Another 1958 survey of 375 randomly selected GPs showed these individuals delivering an average of 8–9 babies per month in their practice (American Academy of General Practice 1958). The 1958 survey also showed GPs performing 11 minor operations and 4 major operations per month on average. AAGP membership data from 1956 reported that over 95 percent of AAGP members provided pediatrics and gynecology services to patients; and over 80 percent provided services in the areas of obstetrics, surgery, proctology, and otolaryngology (American Academy of General Practice 1957).

These figures supported claims the AAGP made in the mid-1950s, using surveys from other stakeholders like Blue Cross Blue Shield insurance plans, that almost all GPs regularly performed surgery, that GPs did approximately 60 percent of all surgical procedures in the United States, and that GPs provided 75 percent of the childcare in the United States (American Academy of General Practice 1958). These types of statistics were meant to assuage the field's fear that their work, the complex kind, was being whittled away by other specialties. A second argument during the 1950s in favor of those believing general practice would remain a going concern was the field's growing membership. In 1955, membership in the American Academy of General Practice, which had only begun as an organization in 1947, reached 20,000 doctors, and they claimed that over 100,000 GPs were working across the United States (American Academy of Family Physicians n.d.).

But the field of general practice was a paper tiger at this point. These statistics belied a deeper malaise, as did the surgical, obstetrics, and pediatrics work GPs still performed during this time. The public was growing enamored with specialty medicine. Technological and scientific advances in medicine, the proliferation of hospitals and academic medical centers, and an embrace after the war of medical specialization produced new medical specialties that grew quickly. Traditional areas of general practice were being taken over by those claiming to be better trained for it, like surgeons. The dollars were flowing to these procedural and niche specialties for research. The proverbial writing was on the wall for general practice. What that meant for the American health care system was a full turn toward a high-cost, sickness-based system of care for patients. A system that narrowly focused procedural specialists would dominate. This meant less attention to improving the health of communities, less attention to the patient holistically and as a unique individual, and a service focus on episodic acute care that treated single illnesses and problems in a vacuum.

General practitioners had an increasingly difficult time gaining hospital privileges during the later 1950s and into the 1960s (American Academy of Family Physicians 1980). This separated them from their sickest patients and undermined their ability to do procedural work like surgery. The issue of hospital privileges for GPs remained front and center for the AAGP every year from the late 1940s onward. As did how GPs should be trained. GP training looked insufficient and haphazard compared to the training for other specialties. Many within the field of general practice felt that GPs should not be engaging in work such as major surgery without better preparation (American Academy of Family Physicians 1980).

The AAGP was not blind to how conditions on the ground were changing. A 1948 AAGP Committee on Education annual report clearly identified the need for general practitioners to work with the American Medical Association (AMA) to improve training for the field (American Academy of General Practice 1948a). It supported the AMA's recommendation of three years of GP residency training beyond medical school, with formal two-year general practice residencies as part of that term. Many in AAGP's leadership knew what was coming if their field did not legitimize itself further through better preparation of its members. The 1948 recommendation included a minimum of one year of training in internal medicine and specialties such as psychiatry, with the second year focusing on obstetrics and pediatrics. Surgical care training was also included in the recommendation, though it was narrowed to focus primarily on training in emergency medicine, postoperative care, and minor surgery. What it specifically spoke against is the GP resident spending significant amounts of residency time working in hospital operating rooms, which effectively preserved major surgical work for the general surgeons and other procedural specialties. This was the first of many times over the next two decades that the field of general practice, and family practice after it, eschewed any form of major procedural work for its members.

A more rigorous residency training experience could not gain significant traction without three things: (a) formal oversight by a general practice specialty certification board, (b) general acceptance of the specific medical knowledge the typical GP needed to learn, and (c) support of other medical specialties who controlled access to the knowledge GPs needed to gain. The suggestion of creating a certification board came up again and again within the general practitioner community, and in the AAGP, through the 1950s and into the 1960s (Young 1995). But it always faced opposition from enough GPs within the AAGP to delay its creation. Some felt it was not needed. Others believed if such a board were created that other medical specialties would end up controlling it, spelling the end of general practice. Still others thought it was a good idea but understood how difficult it would be to enforce and use to improve GP training. This was in part due to long-standing issues with GPs being unable to gain appropriate hospital privileges so that they could have the proper settings in which to train their younger counterparts.

Even as late as 1964, the Congress of Delegates of the AAGP, at their annual meeting, would not vote to support such a board (Pisacano 1970). Yet facts on the ground would not lie. General practice was deteriorating quickly as a viable field of medicine. So it was that during the mid-1960s, the dam protecting traditional general practice could no longer hold. The era of family practice was about to begin.

For specialist physicians in America, there was mostly ambivalence and resistance to a new, better-trained family doctor. These specialties, like neurology, orthopedics, general surgery, pediatrics, and internal medicine, had no problem in the middle part of the twentieth century besmirching the reputation of GPs and taking whatever clinical turf they could from them. Surgeons proactively sought to limit the GP clinical domain. Their professional organization, the American College of Surgeons, had since the 1950s opposed any type of specialty certification for GPs that included major surgical work as part of its accepted work domain (American Academy of Family Physicians 1980). The American College of Physicians, representing general internists, saw general practice as a direct competitor and thus argued in favor of its own members being the overseers of family medicine work. The growing specialty of pediatrics also thought a family medicine specialty might impede on its claim to being the primary care physician for children.

These specialties saw GPs as unfriendly competition. They also had looked down on GPs for a long time because, in their minds, these were doctors who were ill-prepared to practice much of any complex or procedural medicine. General practitioners were not trained like them and had not sacrificed like them. Thus, patients should not believe they were like them. These other specialties had longer, more rigorous residency experiences for their members. They did organized apprenticeships for three years or more versus the typical one-year, ad hoc general practice rotating "internship" that these other fields belittled. Their apprenticeships immersed members in a specific body of medical knowledge. It was unclear what specific knowledge GPs needed to gain during their one internship year. For many of these other doctors, it was a shrug-of-the-shoulders development, holding little value for enhancing their own economic livelihoods or autonomy. In their minds, it had the potential only for harming their own specialties. Organized medicine, think tanks, and government committees could publish as many reports as they wished favoring this notion of the generalist doctor. But in hospitals and doctors' offices across America, most non-GP doctors were having none of it. They knew better.

The 1960s Perfect Storm Calling for a New Comprehensive Physician

If timing is everything, then the 1960s played out for the new specialty of family practice perfectly. The number of doctors self-identifying as general practitioners was in steep decline by the late 1950s. Whereas generalists had outnumbered specialists significantly prior to World War II, with most doctors in the 1930s being generalists, by the 1960s the number of specialists far outpaced the number of general practitioners.

> The general practitioner of revered memory knew his patients, did whatever he could to cure or ease their varied ailments, and provided continuing care through the course of minor ailments and major emergencies. His deficiencies—and they were many—were partly offset by intimate knowledge of his patients, the support he gave them, and the trust and confidence his services engendered. Now he is vanishing. Time has changed both him and his patients. Patients now have access to a richer variety of medical services, and many of them have insurance to help pay for hospital and specialist services.
>
> There are no satisfactory statistics on the number of physicians in general practice. Some physicians who started as general practitioners now limit their practice, wholly or partially, to a specialty, and some with specialty training engage in general practice. There is no doubt, however, that the number and the percentage in general practice are declining. In 1931, 84 percent of all physicians in private practice reported themselves to be general practitioners. In 1960, the corresponding percentage was 45; and in 1965, 37. The percentage is sure to decline further, for of all general practitioners in private practice in 1961, 18 percent were over 65 years of age, a proportion of oldsters much higher than in any other area of practice, and in recent classes of medical school graduates, only

some 15 percent have planned to enter general practice. The general practitioner leaves behind him a vacuum that organized medicine has not decided how to fill. (Millis 1966, pp. 33–34)

By the early 1960s, the label *GP* had acquired many negative connotations. They were considered jacks-of-all-trades, masters-of-none doctors, mostly working in isolation, whose formal preparation and training were seen as, and in most instances were, inferior to that of the super specialists now being churned out by the thousands in medical schools across the country during the 1950s and 1960s. At the same time, the population in America was growing rapidly, with the first of the baby boom generation coming of age as adults and average life spans increasing. More people meant greater need for health care. Particularly primary, preventive, and chronic disease care. The shrinking number of generalist physicians did not align well with that reality. In addition, the mid-1960s saw the establishment of two major government-funded insurance programs, Medicare and Medicaid. Whereas prior to Medicare fewer older Americans had good access to health care services, now they had the backing of the federal government to receive the care they required. Medicaid brought that same access to the poor.

These developments grew demand for a generalist doctor of some kind. They created significant access problems in many parts of the United States that did not have enough doctors. Policy makers also worried more about the affordability of health care in a system that was now dominated by specialists, and which increasingly relied on waiting until people got sick to provide services to them. Family doctors were seen in this regard as potentially efficient, lower-cost professionals to provide less complex care, and preventive services, to American populations.

American society was changing. The relative conformity and quietness of the 1950s gave way to massive upheavals in the 1960s to promote civil rights, social justice, and equality for many traditionally disadvantaged groups of Americans. Grassroots activism was in, and many of these movements gained their fuel from local communities and the champions fighting for change that lived in them. There was a "counterculture" dynamic occurring across many different walks of life. Traditional sources of authority were questioned. Assumptions about "the way things were" were being taken less for granted by many.

The tenor of this time cannot be overstated as an important root cause driving the establishment of a family medicine specialty. There was an opening and leaders of the family medicine movement drove a proverbial truck through it. The questions raised about the viability of a specialty-driven health care system, one too expensive and geared toward the affluent, might not have been uttered without this myriad of developments occurring simultaneously. It gave people reason to question why the system should not be built on a generalist-type physician, and why that physician had been left to wither on the vine.

It was indeed ironic. At the same time the field of general practice was dying, spurned by medical students enamored with technical specialties, conditions on the ground shifted and began screaming out for a kind of comprehensive doctor once again, at least in areas of the country that lacked enough doctors. There was a receptivity, and the intellectual founders of family practice knew it, among key external stakeholders to listen to what this new medical specialty could offer. These stakeholders included powerful physician lobbies like the American Medical Association, state and federal politicians, government agencies, insurance companies, and thousands of small towns and inner cities across the country that lacked enough physicians to provide primary care to a growing insured public.

Several commissioned reports came out at the same time, calling for the need for a family doctor and personal physician who was properly trained and certified, and who could provide first-contact, personalized care for a variety of conditions.* These reports gave justification to push hard for establishing such a specialty. Nicholas Pisacano,† a general

---

* All these reports were published between 1959 and 1966, and all essentially called for a renewed emphasis on primary care in the United States, with a generalist or comprehensive doctor overseeing that form of care delivery. They included the Bane Report, the Willard Committee Report, the Millis Commission Report, and the Folsom Report—major undertakings with sponsorship from powerful professional associations like the AMA and the American Public Health Association.
† We will hear much more from and about Dr. Pisacano, one of the founders of the specialty of family practice.

practitioner in Kentucky who had been writing passionately about the need to create a new, better-trained generalist physician, would become the most ardent early voice for this movement.

The American medical profession, which had moved quickly prior to the 1960s in supporting the growth of new medical specialties (Starr 1982), each focused on specific body parts, organs, or diseases, seemed open in the 1960s, at least on paper, to making family doctors a significant component of the US health care system. The AMA had already passed judgment in the early 1960s on the flailing specialty of general practice, giving it the proverbial kiss of death through its own sponsored Millis Commission Report. This report argued for a new, better-trained army of comprehensive physicians (it did not necessarily support the name *family physicians* yet) to replace the GPs of yesteryear. It also called on the medical training of these new doctors to focus on the comprehensive care needs of patients:

> A much more sweeping change is necessary. Continuing, comprehensive care should be a central focus of medical school organization, planning, and clinical teaching. Right at the beginning of the student's introduction to clinical medicine he should begin to realize, and his teachers should emphasize, that illness is usually not an isolated event in a localized part of the body, but is a change in a complex, integrated human being who lives and works in a particular social and family setting, who has a biological-psychological-social history. . . . The good primary physicians now in practice have acquired much of their skill and wisdom from experience, or from intuition. What is needed and what the medical schools and teaching hospitals must try to develop is a body of information and general principles concerning man as a whole and man in society that will provide an intellectual framework into which the lessons of practical experience can be fitted. This background will be partly biological, but partly it will be social and humanistic, for it will deal with man as a total, complex, integrated social being. (Millis 1966, pp. 45, 51)

The AMA had not necessarily intended to focus on producing a report that would call specifically for a new version of the generalist physician. After all, the Millis Report had the larger goal of looking at how to reform and make appropriate changes to medical education and training generally. The reality was that in practice, the AMA busied itself for years on selling the outside world on the idea of a fragmented, highly technical, super-specialized version of medicine. First, because it meant greater prestige and collective power accorded to the medical profession (Starr 1982), and second, because with this prestige and power would come greater economic rewards for all doctors throughout the medical profession.

Two professional associations already representing doctors in primary care, the American College of Physicians representing internists and the American Association of Pediatrics, opposed a new family medicine specialty. Each group felt it could provide this new comprehensive care delivery. But despite this opposition among key professional organizations, the AMA came around to the side of family medicine. The AMA was under increased pressure to support ways of expanding patient access to more doctors, ones who were also as well trained in their respective fields as possible. It saw an opportunity in expanding the reach of primary care medicine into areas of the country where access to any kind of doctor was problematic, and in focusing on a brand of physician with the goal of prevention and keeping people healthy. The AMA's Millis Report again weighed in on this:

> Despite the rising expectations and rising usage of medical services, there are unrecognized and unmet needs. . . . Rural residents, persons with little means, members of some ethnic groups, and some of the institutionalized patients receive less medical care than do more fortunate citizens. Leaders of medicine share with other leaders of the country a vision of greater future possibilities, of more widespread and more effective preventive care, of health protection as well as the cure of disease. . . . The continuing rise in expectations and demands must surely affect the educational needs of future physicians. (Millis 1966, pp. 23–24)

As the 1960s moved forward, the general idea of providing each patient with a doctor who could coordinate all their needs and make them healthier had value. Not only for continuing to advance the medical profession's power, but for growing the younger procedural specialties* that could use family doctors as conduits for accessing their own more expensive services. It was an idea that resonated with people's sense of what medicine could be from a human rather than technical perspective. A kind, empathic, interpersonal brand of healing that maintained some of the traditional romanticized view of the doctor that modern procedural medicine in many ways undermined. Family practice could offer a good sales pitch in this way to a lot of different stakeholders. But it would also serve as a feeder for higher-cost medicine.

Who could argue with a doctor whose primary focus was on "the family" in American society? Who was against family? It was not only something the public needed practically and wanted in the abstract. It was something that could strengthen medicine's grip on health care in the United States. It could enhance their overall brand with the public. While the AMA may have at first been brought around somewhat reluctantly to supporting a new generalist physician specialty, there was strategic value to be realized for the entire profession in doing so. Yes, even for the internists and pediatricians who opposed it.

Nick Pisacano's Crusade and the Final Nail in the General Practice Coffin

Support aside, was it a radical and innovative idea, this notion of having a better-trained comprehensive family doctor to replace the general practitioner? The answer to that question might depend on who you asked during the 1960s. Certainly, those individuals at the forefront of the movement in the 1960s believed it to be so. Nick Pisacano thought it radical and innovative, both in terms of the potential scope of the new specialty, which would be even more focused on community health and longitudinal care and prevention for patients, and the rigorous extent to which the new family doctors could be trained to do their jobs. Others

---

* A *procedural* medical specialty is just that—a specialty in which the doctors focus on performing procedures on patients.

agreed with him. Many of them, active general practitioners later in their careers, had a vested personal interest in advocating for a stronger version of themselves. For these doctors, a new and improved primary care specialty was music to their ears. They had lived with hearing the negativity associated with the GP label, and they knew that a fresh name and formal training system that could weed out poorly trained family doctors could help legitimize their own competency in the role.

Much of the public, particularly in areas where physicians were scarce, continued to use general practitioners in the 1960s and relied on them for their care, like the citizens of Fayette, Alabama, where Richard Rutland worked. For these Americans, the GP was the physician with whom they were most familiar, and perhaps the only doctor with whom they came into contact in a given year. Doctors like Richard Rutland. In addition, millions of poor and elderly Americans who now had insurance coverage through Medicaid and Medicare wanted to see a doctor and receive care. For them, a new specialty focused on holistic and family care delivery, in addition to basic primary care and chronic disease management, was a no-brainer.

Prior to 1960 nobody besides a small band of advocates had pushed seriously for a dedicated and highly qualified generalist branch of medicine, properly blessed by the entire medical profession, in which the doctors in theory could be (a) the first contact for patients needing the health care system; (b) responsible for coordinating the total needs of patients across the life span, that is, as care managers; (c) caring for entire families; and (d) contributors to the health of the larger community in which they lived. But there were true believers that would not give up, and Dr. Nicholas Pisacano was their leader.

Nick Pisacano was born in Philadelphia on June 6, 1924, and raised in Merchantville, New Jersey. He was called a Renaissance man by his peers. A physician-intellectual, yet a pragmatist who sought to take on the medical status quo. A street fighter underneath philosopher garb. World War II veteran, sports-lover, skilled pianist, reader of Latin and Greek classic literature, and avid book collector, he worked diligently to bring people around to his point of view. He did not mince words. For example, in 1989, a year before his death, when the idea of merging the specialties of internal medicine and family medicine into one specialty was presented to him, he replied, "I'm telling you we will not merge the two specialties as long as I can breathe" (*Canadian Family Physician* 1989).

The man who founded the American Board of Family Medicine (ABFM) in 1969 and served as its chief intellectual leader until his death in 1990, and who founded the *Journal of the American Board of Family Practice,* the flagship academic outlet for the ABFM, was a general practitioner who had practiced in both rural and urban areas during the 1950s and early 1960s. In the 1960s he dedicated himself to a career in academic medicine at the University of Kentucky Medical Center. It was here where he established one of the first family medicine residency programs, where he became a highly popular professor with his students, and where he would spend his entire career (*Journal of the American Medical Association* 1990). A lifelong friend of his commented upon his death:

> Nick lived not only an active and passionate life, but a carefully examined one. He loved and hated with equal fervor. . . . He had a lifelong romance with books and literature, which he shared with all of us. He could quote endlessly from such disparate sources as the Bible and Henry Mencken. He loved music and the arts and reveled in his Roman heritage. He suffered no fools but had tireless patience for the young, the ill, and the mistreated. Beneath the carefully cultivated gruff exterior . . . lived a warm and tender Nickie, who believed disease and poverty were crimes against humanity and wanted desperately to eliminate them. He ran out of time. (Hamburg 1990)

Pisacano is central to this part of the story of family medicine because there was no single person more important to the birth of the new specialty. He assumed this leadership role with relish. In 1964, in the pages of *General Practice,* the flagship journal of the American Academy of General Practice, he called for the destruction of traditional general practice in advance of the new specialty of family practice.

> Most of us now recognize that the species of physicians known as the general practitioner is all but extinct. A few of these creatures are still about the country, but for all practical purposes, the real old-fashioned general practitioner is now a glorious subject for a chapter in the text-

books of medical history. He was the vital force in American medicine when he flourished. No type of physician surpassed him in having general all-around ability to diagnose and treat the ills of his patients, as well as having a personal knowledge of his families in their own setting, their problems and interrelationships among themselves and with the community. Enough praise could never be heaped in such a short dissertation as this on behalf of the old general practitioner, but I come to bury him, not to praise him. (Pisacano 1964, p. 173)

When you purposefully cast something as dead or dying, you hopefully have something else in mind to take its place. For Pisacano, this was a family practice specialty. There had always been a family medicine faction within the larger specialty of general practice, and it agitated for this new specialty, but it had not gained significant traction as of the early 1960s. For example, during the early 1960s handfuls of GPs attempted to create a specialty of family practice through the establishment of a new oversight board and a three-year residency program, but their efforts were rebuffed by the larger American Academy of General Practice. There had also been ongoing but unsuccessful attempts within the AAGP, beginning in the early 1950s, to change its name to the American Academy of Family Physicians.

It could be said that the larger field of general practice was ambivalent about the whole idea, frightened by what a family practice specialty might mean for its survival. They realized that it likely meant the death of the specialty in its current form, and that it would create problems for many of its members. Even into the 1960s, with the winds of change blowing against them, the AAGP still tried to contain the family medicine movement within its own body, listening to its desires but demurring on taking any significant action.

In 1966, in collaboration with the AMA Section on General Practice, the AAGP produced a document entitled, "The Core Content of Family Medicine,"* which was published in its flagship journal (American

* Each medical specialty has a "core content" document that articulates the specific knowledge and competencies associated with being a "qualified" doctor in that given specialty.

Academy of General Practice 1966). This document stated the myriad responsibilities and activities encompassed by the field of family medicine, including, but not limited to, preventive medicine, relational care delivery, diagnosis, treatment and management, end-of-life and geriatric care, family counseling, and community medicine. Clinging steadfastly to the label of *general practitioner*, the AAGP nonetheless was trying desperately to keep the budding family medicine movement within its organizational confines, and within the work and responsibilities of the traditional general practitioner in America. It also was responding to the recent submission of a specialty board certification application for family practice, supported by Pisacano and others, which had been rejected once by the American Board of Medical Specialties but which, given the recent reports published advocating for a comprehensive medicine specialty, was gaining traction within the medical profession.*

There were many GPs in America neither trained adequately enough to become this new type of family doctor or able to do the full scope of work outlined in the AAGP's core content document in a competent manner. Many GPs feared both the potential competition of this new breed of family doctor and what it might mean for their livelihoods and careers. Especially if they were suddenly asked to retrain or go through an arduous certification process—which was Pisacano's strong preference if the new family practice doctor was to have credibility. There were many GPs who had practiced in their little corner of the world for years. They had been unbothered by stricter licensing or board certification requirements, happily continuing to perform surgeries, deliver babies, and do all sorts of diverse care delivery, even as surgical and obstetric specialties grew around them. For these GPs, a family medicine specialty was unnecessary and a potential threat to their own position in the status quo.

---

* The American Board of Medical Specialties, in cooperation with the American Medical Association, has the authority to approve "specialty boards" for each medical specialty. The specialty boards serve as the formal oversight for intellectual content within a given specialty and administer qualifying exams to doctors interested in getting licensed in that specialty.

There is little doubt that there were already other general practitioners, particularly in rural America, that performed with competence the wider range of functions associated with a new family medicine specialty. They had been doing so for some time. Like Richard Rutland, they had years and often decades of experience performing all aspects of comprehensive primary care medicine. They would be the equal if not the superior of any new family medicine physicians produced under a more rigorous training system. For these GPs, it was more a matter of semantics since their everyday work would not change. At most, it would help their careers and self-esteem. But these doctors would need assurance that they could earn the new label of *family physician* without an overly onerous path to gaining that recognition.

By 1966, time was running out. In a paper published that year entitled "Family Practice as a Specialty," Pisacano summarized a dire situation:

> The decline in general practice has been very great. In 1931, there were
> 112,000 general practitioners; in 1964, the figure stood at 67,000. . . .
> Many students believe that the broad body of knowledge required for
> family practice is too great; some fear for lack of prestige; lack of exposure
> to family physicians in the standard four-year medical school curriculum
> and, conversely, constant contact with specialists in medical schools serve
> as recruiting mechanisms for specialties. Family doctors are finding it
> more difficult than ever to get hospital privileges in community hospitals.
> This deprivation of privileges is probably because increasing numbers of
> fair-sized hospitals are requiring their staff members to be board certified
> or board qualified in some specialty. . . . The most important factor in the
> opinion of this author is that the general practitioner of the past can no
> longer be all things to all people. . . . As far as image, many students
> believe the family doctor not only lacks status professionally but also
> fares poorly in the eyes of the public. (Pisacano 1966, pp. 12–14)

Nick Pisacano had taken to using the term *family doctor* even as he was referring to the traditional general practitioner. In this way he was already moving on his and others' idea for creating a new primary care specialty. His take was dead on. Few young medical students wanted to become general practitioners in the 1960s. It simply held little allure next to the glitz and glamor of higher-paying specialties that were connected to the new academic medical centers. Many young students smart enough to earn their way into medical school were also interested in the science of clinical research and studying medical problems on an abstract and intellectual level as well as doing direct patient care. They wanted to lend their talents to a smaller yet highly specific and technical body of work versus the broader, more abstract work of the general practitioner. As he noted, the age of specialization in medicine had arrived, and it held appeal to lots of very bright, motivated young medical students.

By the mid-1960s, it was a foregone conclusion that the formal training to become a general practitioner left something to be desired and was out of step with the rest of American medicine. Traditionally, most GPs did a year-long rotating internship after medical school where they would ideally gain exposure to various areas of clinical practice, including surgery and obstetrics. But these internships were highly varied across the country in terms of quality and content. If you saw one GP internship, you saw one GP internship. In the early 1960s, there was an attempt to create two-year GP internships. But this experiment failed because there was still little quality control over them, and no one could agree on what should be in them.

Whereas the field of general practice in 1949 had less than 20 percent of its more than 9,100 internship positions left vacant, by 1965 less than 50 percent of general practice residency slots were filled, and by 1967 only 132 of 824 (16 percent) available GP training slots were being filled (Rodnick 1987; Stephens 2010). The field was dying. In Pisacano's mind, that was fine, because he believed that GP residency experiences were grossly insufficient to produce a competent family doctor anyway. Better to have them sit empty than fill them with young physicians who would not get the appropriate training to be true family doctors. Better to let the end come quickly.

For the generalist physician community, there were going to be winners and losers in the development of a viable family practice specialty, particularly given the widespread support for making the requirements to enter into that new specialty high, and similar to the requirements for other clinical fields. The losers would be those GPs not adequately trained to perform the role in the manner envisioned by the Millis Report and leaders like Pisacano. GPs who would neither be willing or able to retrain themselves formally to meet the new standards of the comprehensive doctor. GPs who would view this requirement as a personal insult to their years of experience and dedication to the craft of general practice. The winners would be GPs like Richard Rutland, already well-trained and experienced, who would not be intimidated or put off by any new requirements for practice; GPs who saw in the development of a family practice specialty an opportunity to gain greater acceptance with patients and their specialist colleagues; and GPs who saw an opportunity to expand their responsibilities, and hopefully get more recognition for it, in ways that were personally satisfying to them.

Regardless of how many GPs fell on one side of the argument and how many on the other, one thing became clear to people like Pisacano as discussions around a family practice specialty became more serious as the 1960s rolled on. The traditional notion of the poorly trained general practitioner would have to be destroyed completely if possible. There could be no way for this new specialty to be confused with the old one, or for the baggage associated with the old specialty to undermine this new one. This was one of the prices for evolving the concept of the comprehensive doctor in a way that gained it wide acceptance, especially within the confines of organized medicine. The American Academy of General Practice and its leadership during the 1950s and early 1960s had always known this fact, which is why they had resisted it for so long. It was a price Pisacano and many of his generalist colleagues thought fair, necessary, and overdue. Yet it was a price that once paid would heighten the expectations everyone had for this new specialty, placing it into a difficult position moving forward for years to come.

The new family practice specialty would need to sever from the *general practitioner* label and its rich, anachronistic history fully and unapologetically. It would do so by casting general practice as deficient in knowledge and training, and by casting family practice as a sophisticated, deep, and diverse field of medicine. It would define family practice as a field that could deliver many things to many people, and the family doctor as an uber-doctor of the noblest order. In this way those like Nick Pisacano intended to cleanse people's minds of the GP label and put the final nail in the coffin of a type of physician that for many was no longer acceptable. It would be a general practitioner that led this charge.

But words would not be enough. There needed to be a strategy to support the ascendance of family practice in America. Pisacano and others had one in mind. That strategy was multifaceted and relied on imitating other medical specialties, a grandiose yet noncontroversial definition for what family doctors would do, and trying to sell the notion of a generalist doctor who was also a "specialist" like all other doctors. A strategy that was bold as well as conformist, yet one whose early victories would be paid for later with a string of defeats that would leave family practice at the mercy of a hostile health care system.

June 25, 1997

Dear Dr. Rutland,

Please tell me it ain't so! You have always been there for me and my family. "Thank you" seems so inadequate. I was only about 6 or 7 when first I was seen in your office; and now I am a very mature 50 year old woman. You have been there through the births of my two girls, Tami and Melanie, and our recent loss of Daddy in January.

I wanted to tell you a funny little story about the time you were in the "Good Housekeeping" magazine—when you were selected as the "Physician of the Year." I was living in Connecticut at the time; Claude was still in the Navy. I had been to the grocery store that day—I almost never purchased magazines, but something just made me buy the "Good Housekeeping" magazine that day. I had to wait until late that night to look at it. There I was in the bed with all my family asleep, and I am turning pages in the magazine and come across this picture. I looked at it and thought to myself, "hmm, that looks like somebody I know." So I got out of bed and went to the kitchen to get a better look—and there is my doctor, dear Dr. Rutland, in the magazine! I was so overcome and so loud I awoke my entire family. Of course, they all wanted to know what was the matter with me; and when I told them, they just looked at me with disgust, turned, and went back to bed. Anyway, the next day I took it to work and showed everyone.

What a wonderful doctor and friend you have been to Fayette County! Many thanks to your patient and kind family in allowing us to have your services at your clinic and at the hospital. I know you missed many, many things with your family due to your devotion to your profession.

May your retirement be as fulfilling as your years of service as a doctor.

Lauren A.

Patient letter to Dr. Rutland upon his retirement, 1997 (Rutland Papers, Center for the History of Family Medicine)

FIVE

Saying Hello to the New and Improved Family Doctor

IN THE SAME 1966 paper where he cut to the chase about the decline of general practice among medical students, Dr. Nicholas Pisacano waxed philosophical regarding the definition of a new family practice specialty, laying the groundwork for the training focus and requirements he and others saw as integral to meeting this ideal.

> Administrators and educators repeatedly have been asking us to define Family Practice. Family Practice has to be defined in two ways. First, a functional definition: Family Practice is a method of practice. It is not limited to an organ system nor is it limited to an age group. One does Family Practice; one does not study it. . . . Let us propose then, this general, overall description: Family Practice is, literally, the quintessence of Medicine. The prime essence of Internal Medicine plus the secondary essence, Pediatrics; the third and fourth essences of Psychiatry and Community Medicine. Family Practice, then, is the fifth essence or quintessence which interrelates the other four essences, whose total is greater than their sum by virtue of its integrative function and application to the social unit we call the family.
> (Pisacano 1966, pp. 15–16)

Quintessence of medicine? Now that is one way to try and sell what you do—and a mouthful to be sure. But while Pisacano's positioning of family practice as the most comprehensive and diverse branch of medicine was rhetorically grand, it was also pragmatic and strategic, as it allowed family practice to stake a claim to specific knowledge already claimed by four other medical specialties. If anyone had a doubt as to who could provide the care these other specialties laid claim to, or what exactly the modern family doctor should be concerned with, Pisacano left no room for interpretation in his 1964 eulogy paper:

> The answer is the family doctor! This means the birth of the specialty of family practice, the production of adequately and properly trained family doctors. We do not mean a spottily-trained graduate with a smattering of all disciplines who becomes a general practitioner, neither do we mean a specialty trained internist who has little or no training in the areas outside of internal medicine.
>
> The true family doctor should handle capably and completely minor surgical procedures, well babies, sick babies and minor illnesses without bemoaning the nonserious nature of the disease. He should listen to the psychoneurotic with patience and sensitivity and guide him properly without contempt; he should render diagnostic and therapeutic measures for the common gynecologic disorders, especially in cancer detection; he should treat properly the very omnipresent ear, nose and throat disorders, and besides this, with his training broadly and solidly based in internal medicine, he should manage many of the "major" hospital illnesses. Most important, he should counsel the family in health matters, treat the patient when he can or maintain liaison with the specialist to whom he has referred the patient. He should relate the illness not only to the patient and the family, but to the community, utilizing his knowledge of community medicine in its broadest sense. When any physician assumes this concept of family care, then, and only then, should he call himself a family doctor. (Pisacano 1964, p. 175)

The amount of paper spent on defining family practice and the role of the family doctor during the 1960s could fill several volumes on a shelf. And it all flowed from Pisacano's swing-for-the-fences definition.

All these definitions in some form included the responsibilities he placed on the new family doctor's turf. Responsibilities such as care management, community health, relational care for individuals and families, preventive care, basic acute care, care coordination, and providing guidance to patients. Much of this work was little different from how the field of general practice had defined itself for years prior, including in its "Core Content of Family Medicine" published in 1966 and discussed in the previous chapter (American Academy of General Practice 1966). What was different was that Pisacano and others believed that with the proper training and support, the new family doctor could do all of it very well.

The training system for general practitioners (GPs) was grossly inadequate in his eyes. He sought a definition that would please the rest of organized medicine and satisfy societal needs for the kind of doctor outlined in the Millis Report and others. But make no mistake. It would be a well-prepared and capable doctor who, at the same time, did not seek to do significant surgical or procedural work—a line of work GPs had seen wither over time and the emerging specialties take over. A line of work that would have brought family practice into immediate conflict with these other specialties. No, the family physician would not be a high-level technician like those in other specialties.

For example, nowhere in Pisacano's definition did it claim that family doctors should be meaningfully invested in delivering babies—something which many general practitioners still did on a regular basis. It identified only "minor" surgical procedures as appropriate, which implied simple tasks like stitching up a small cut, but not anything more serious or procedural in nature. This was music to the ears of the surgical specialties. It was also consistent with the "Essentials for Residency Training in Family Practice" that the American Medical Association House of Delegates had approved in December 1968, and which Pisacano's rhetoric had influenced. In those essentials, there was little mention of significant training in any procedural area that would conflict with other doctors like gynecologists or surgeons.

With respect to surgery, for example, the "Essentials" document stated that "The [family practice] resident should acquire competence in recognizing surgical emergencies and when appropriate referring them for necessary specialized care" and "He should be trained in basic surgical principles by recognized surgical specialists and acquire from them the technical proficiency required to manage those limited surgical procedures a first contact [family] physician may be called upon to perform. If he expects to include major surgery as part of his regular practice, he should obtain additional training" (American Medical Association 1968). In other words, the family practice resident would not learn how to perform major surgical work because it would not be part of their everyday job. If they wanted to do any type of major surgery, they needed to engage in the specific residency training that aspiring surgeons completed. Pisacano's definition instead made the family doctor, by necessity, a professional who needed to coordinate the work of a patient's other doctors. Someone serving as the manager of their care needs but also their first-level diagnostician—a tricky job when there was a lot of clinical turf that could not be treaded upon. The Millis Report (1966) had staked out a similar focus for the new family doctor:

> We suggest that he be called a primary physician. He should usually be primary in the first-contact sense. He will serve as the primary medical resource and counselor to an individual or a family. When a patient needs hospitalization, the services of other medical specialists, or other medical or paramedical assistance, the primary physician will see that the necessary arrangements are made, giving such responsibility to others as is appropriate, and retaining his own continuing and comprehensive responsibility. (Millis 1966, p. 37)

The Challenges of an Opaque, Wide-Ranging Definition of the Family Doctor

The approach Nick Pisacano and his colleagues chose was a smart one in a short-term, strategic way. They sought to allay the concerns of other medical specialties that family medicine would encroach on their turf, while at the same time conveying a sense of mutually beneficial partnership with those specialties. *We are your partners, not your competitors,* was the mantra. *We can help you, and make sure the right patient business comes to you easier.* In return, Pisacano wanted the new family doctor recognized as the type of doctor most able and willing to develop ongoing relationships with patients and entire families. He wanted them to act as the overseers of people's care. In his mind, that would give this new doctor an essential role in the lives of patients and in their communities, even if that role would be very difficult to perform in reality.

In this unique moment of time during the late 1960s, when the conditions seemed perfect for pushing the field of family practice, this was the positioning suggested for this new brand of doctor. These opaque definitions of family practice became the foundation for subsequent definitions put forth over the next several decades, with only slight semantic enhancements, such as the family physician serving as "first contact care" and providing "care coordination" for patients. Consider this almost identical definition to Pisacano's 1964 one that was put forth fifty years later by a working group organized by the American Academy of Family Physicians and charged with clarifying the definition of family medicine in the modern age:

> Family physicians are personal doctors for people of all ages and health
> conditions. They are a reliable first contact for health concerns and
> directly address most health care needs. Through enduring partnerships,
> family physicians help patients prevent, understand, and manage illness,
> navigate the health system and set health goals. Family physicians and their
> staff adapt their care to the unique needs of their patients and communities.
> They use data to monitor and manage their patient population and use
> best science to prioritize services most likely to benefit health. They are
> ideal leaders of health care systems and partners for public health. (Phillips
> et al. 2014)

Many of the intellectual leaders of the family medicine movement from the 1970s through the 2000s would end up writing about the enduring problem of pitching family doctors this way. No doubt, early proponents of a family practice specialty like Nick Pisacano were trying to have it both ways. They wanted to create a family doctor identity that sounded highly prestigious and universally helpful, one that would appeal to patients, policy makers, and the medical profession. But at the same time, they wanted to be vague about the specific scope of work family doctors would perform to avoid angering certain stakeholders in or out of the profession (but especially inside) whose interests could be negatively affected by a definition that outlined specific work already claimed by other specialties.

Unfortunately, these definitions of family practice and the family doctor would prove problematic over time. They would create ambiguity and confusion in the minds of some family doctors as to "the right way" to fulfill their roles and enact their careers. They would lead to ambivalence in the minds of the public, policy makers, and the medical profession itself—none of whom would ever truly understand what exactly it was a family doctor was supposed to do and to what extent. But an even greater problem was that the notion of an expansive, opaque role for family doctors, one that centered on managing a patient's comprehensive care needs, made it an impossible job to do fully or well. It would be a job too dependent on the availability of services in the larger community and the individual patient's own ability and interest to play along. It needed fair compensation from insurers, who were not willing to pay for it. It needed patients who could be followed over time and who were very engaged in their own care. And it required a lot of time, effort, and knowledge on the part of family doctors, even as they would be paid much less than other doctors. It would not be the glamorous procedural work other specialties did to earn higher prestige and pay. It would be a lot of thankless grunt work whose end results might take years to see in some patient situations.

Who could do all this? Who would want to for long periods of their careers, especially when the rewards of the work were often unseen for long periods of time? When the rest of the health care system did not really support it? Why would the rest of organized medicine allow one specialty to have such far-flung, vague powers over American health care and patients? Despite these unanswered questions, Pisacano continued to push the notion of a family doctor in the role of comprehensive care overseer.

This particular primary physician assumes the total responsibility for the care and health needs of that patient and his family. He refers when necessary, but he takes care of these people when he can—when he knows he can handle them. He assesses their total needs and provides these needs according to his training and his ability. But, in contrast with other primary physicians, he takes on comprehensive care. . . . He assumes the comprehensive and continuous care of this patient and/or his family. (Pisacano 1970)

To achieve Pisacano's ideal of a comprehensive care overseer, family doctors were expected to perform a number of duties: care coordinator, care manager, full-scope diagnostician, health care intellectual, critical thinker for patients, community advocate and social justice pursuer, holder of all patient information deemed important for health, representative for all of health care, and relational bond between patients and the health care system. But a single human who can fulfill all these duties to the letter has not yet been built. Would it be great to have a single doctor who could do all this for the same large number of patients over the course of twenty or thirty years? Absolutely. The image of the wise, all-knowing general doctor, understanding and empathetic, available day or night, is the reason *Marcus Welby, M.D.* was the number one television show in America in 1970, and why we continue to be fascinated with watching shows and reading personal testimonials about doctors and what they do.

But has it ever been a realistic expectation for a single physician? Sure, general practitioners like Dr. Richard Rutland had been playing multiple roles for the better part of their careers. But he performed some of these roles more than others, for a smaller community and group of patients, and in the personal context of giving up much of his own life to try and get it done. He was also working within a health system that, in the 1950s and 1960s, was under the direct control of the doctor. It was a health care system without the interference of insurance companies and government programs like Medicare, without the burden of needing to document everything done on each patient to get paid and having to do tons of paperwork to get needed services and medications approved for patients, and without powerful specialists on every American street corner making their services available directly to patients. Doctors coming after Rutland in the 1970s and beyond would not be so lucky, would not have as much opportunity, and would not want to give up huge chunks of themselves to fulfill the promise of the family doctor ideal, as we will soon see.

Old Wine in Better Looking Skins? Selling Family Practice as a New "Specialty"

The problems with the definitional approach Pisacano and others took were either not well understood at the time or ignored for the short-term benefits the effective marketing of that definition could bring to legitimizing the new family doctor. It was a deal with the devil. For the definitional issue would arguably hinder rather than enhance the field's ability to gain public and professional acceptance over time. It would lead family doctors, like their general practitioner forebearers, to be perceived as better trained but still jacks-of-all-trades, masters of none. It would not raise the prestige of the generalist doctor in hoped-for ways, nor lead to a fundamental transformation of the health care system toward primary care and keeping people healthy. It would not stop the continued financial devaluing of some primary care services like care management. Such services would remain difficult to perform, vague, invisible to most stakeholders, and thus unable to convince the public and insurers of their worth.

It would also lead to a challenging identity for family doctors to embrace. It would confuse both current and prospective family doctors by making many of them wonder, on an everyday basis, what they were supposed to be doing, and how exactly they were supposed to do it all in a hostile health care system. It would make them question the notion that the definition itself implied—that the only right way to be a family doctor was to be a full-time outpatient medicine clinician, hunkered down in one geographic place for a long time, and working with the same patients over years to get to know them in order to provide all of these management, advisory, and coordination services. What if some family doctors did not want to do this? Could they still be family doctors? Would they be accepted? Was it worth becoming a family doctor if they were not sure they could fulfill the role in the manner Pisacano and others wanted?

Additionally, the new family doctor could and should, according to these definitions, also situate themselves squarely in the community in which they lived—learning about and knowing how that community promoted or undermined their patients' health. To be an effective patient advocate and care manager, to gain the respect of other physician colleagues, and to cultivate patient relationships, it was critical to embed oneself in the local community, like the country doctor of yore, like Richard Rutland—only with better training.

> We have included [in family practice training] the unique discipline of Community Medicine. This, of course, stresses the principles of epidemiology and environmental health, and a general understanding of the health resources in that community. We like our physician to know what the community is all about—everything about the community. Is it a sick community? Is it a healthy community? What are its needs? Just as you would look at a patient. (Pisacano 1970)

Perhaps this intent was the most ambitious part of the entire definition: the idea that the family doctor was supposed to be a difference maker for patients by practicing "community medicine"—understanding the local community's health status, getting involved in local efforts to improve public health, and raising patients' awareness of how their surroundings might affect their health. While the field of general practice might claim to have always been interested in this set of activities, and doctors like Rutland engaged in them as needed, in the eyes of Pisacano each new family doctor should hold themselves personally accountable for making sure they walked this walk.

It was a gamble to push a family practice specialty in this way, to put the older wine of the well-rounded general practitioner into newer skins. Skins that convinced the outside world of the superiority of the new family doctor. These were not roles and responsibilities in which the family doctor would dabble or pick and choose. They were to be trained properly to do every one of them. It would be the essence of the family doctor's identity and everyday work, and it was a big bet to make. Would the public, insurance companies paying the bills, and other clinical specialties buy on faith, at least at the outset, that activities like care management or gatekeeping were good for them? Would they view these roles positively? Would they be able to understand what they entailed? Could these services be specific and valued enough to ascribe specific financial value to them? Could everyone give up the necessary control to family doctors so that they could be comprehensive physicians? These questions would hound family practice throughout its fifty-year existence.

Another part of the gamble was one that Pisacano and his ilk saw clearly and sought to head off from the outset. There was the risk that the public, especially, but also young 1960s medical students turning away from general practice as a career in droves, and those entering medical school in the future, might not see this incarnation of the new family doctor as anything dramatically different from what was there before. To address this head-on, the new family doctor would be sold as another type of "specialist," since that word held magical value in the American lexicon in the 1960s.

> Essentially, the task of this new physician is to exemplify all of medicine to the patient. He will be a specialist in family medicine; but in certain crucial aspects, the new "family physician" will differ from all other specialists. His specialty will not be based on organs or organ systems, age groups, operational procedures, treatment modalities or disease entities—categories that embrace most if not all the presently recognized clinical specialties. Instead, this new physician's special calling will be based on function—on the care and management of whole patients, and patients contemplated in the context of their families, homes, jobs and personal histories. He will be first and foremost a diagnostician, utilizing all the technical and professional aides available to help him.
>
> A second radical distinction of the new family physician is that he will be a specialist by inclusion—in contrast to the classical clinical specialist who specializes by excluding. His aim is to broaden his concern, to widen his skill; he seeks to accept responsibility; not merely

to pass it along. He utilizes specialists, rather than surrendering to them. The new physician, because of the breadth of his function and range of his concern, will be a director, rather than a doer—a manager rather than a technician. Like his counterpart in industry, he will delegate every conceivable operational task to his aides. He will make the so-called "health team" an operating reality, rather than the rhetorical fantasy that it is today. (Family Health Foundation of America 1969, pp. 33–34)

Of course, the embodiment of the family doctor as a "specialist" remained rooted in the complex, all-consuming generalist role Pisacano had staked out. The term *specialist* had already gained a connotation in American society, and in the medical profession. It was someone who knew a lot about a little, whose duties were highly technical and narrowly defined. Pisacano and the family practice advocates wanted to co-opt the term to brand family doctors in a favorable way to the outside world. They thought that by using this label they could create the perception that family doctors deserved a rightful place alongside the orthopedist, internist, and other medical specialists. They really did believe that the scientific content of family medicine was "specialized" in the sense of its rigor and uniqueness. But it was still a generalist role.

Seeking not only to co-opt but to confuse the very definition of the term was a genius move early on. It could help shift the preferred identity of family doctors away from general practitioners without anyone noticing too much. It could move that identity closer to other types of better trained doctors in a way that was noncontroversial, particularly to these other doctors, since the work of the family doctor would remain non-procedural in nature. Most ambitiously, it could perhaps help set the stage for a total reconceptualization of the word *specialty* in American medicine. Maybe. Family doctors would be specialists in terms of the breadth of medical knowledge they possessed and the comprehensive attention they gave to the health needs of the entire person and larger family unit. They would know a lot about a lot, not a lot about a little. According to Pisacano, the "medicine" in family medicine would not be narrow but expansive. It would require a significant formal structure to support it, so it justified the imitation approach to training that was also being proposed for family doctors. Speaking in 1970 about the effort undertaken to brand family doctors as specialists, he noted:

> We established three criteria. We felt (a) that family practice is a specialty; (b) as a specialty it deserves graduate training programs; and (c) that those who pursue and fulfill the graduate training requirements should be certified. . . . In contrast with other primary physicians, he takes on comprehensive care, and therein, I think, lies the difference between other primary physicians and our particularly primary physician. . . . The length of graduate training is three years after the attainment of the medical degree. . . . I happen to be one of those physicians who believes that the heart of all medicine is internal medicine. And we do weigh internal medicine heavily in our three year program. We also include pediatrics. We have included in our program psychiatry. . . . We want them to have a good understanding of the biological and psychosocial aspects of pregnancy, ante-partum and post-partum care, and non-operative obstetrics in general. We want our man to be adept at so-called "medical" or "office" gynecology. (Pisacano 1970)

Again, family doctors would be trained to understand the medicine of several different medical specialties, but they would not be *proceduralists* in any sense of the term, like other clinical specialties. Because, as we have seen, the definition of family practice Pisacano and others put forth discouraged almost any kind of procedural medicine. But just calling oneself a specialty does not make it so. By defining family practice work away from performing procedures, and away from settings like the hospital, the early leaders of the movement turned a blind eye to what many of its prospective members were already doing in the real world. Comprehensive primary care for many general practitioners and new family medicine recruits of the time meant the work of delivering babies and regularly doing procedures like sigmoidoscopies.* It also

---

* A sigmoidoscopy is a procedure where a doctor inserts a flexible, lighted tube up and into a patient's sigmoid colon looking for abnormal growths or ulcers.

meant seeing patients in the hospital and in emergency rooms every day, being a key part of the complex clinical work done in those settings.

As noted, carving out most of the technical aspects of medicine and leaving them to other specialties was part of the short-term bargain Pisacano and the early founders made to gain support for family practice. Yet it would undermine the attractiveness and perception of the field moving forward. It would make family doctoring look like a thankless job at times, where doctors were trying to control things outside of any single doctor's control. It created the perception of a job loaded with administrative tasks and insurance paperwork, without any of the glitz and glamour of immediately saving a life or fixing an important clinical problem quickly and in an exciting way. It would also hinder any acceptance of this specialty as a co-equal of other medical specialties where a scalpel or sophisticated tool was used regularly on patients.

It would help allow gynecologists, a competing group of doctors, to pitch themselves as the primary care doctors for women of childbearing age. It would open the door for other new specialties to arise in the 1970s and late 1990s, such as emergency medicine and hospital medicine—who were only too eager to occupy themselves with a small area of medicine rather than a comprehensive one. Pisacano and others certainly believed they could sell family medicine as a specialty focused on patient management and generalist care delivery. But what if few others bought into that vision? This led to another part of the strategy—to try and make family practice look like every other specialty in terms of the training and certification process.

Repackaging and Imitation to Gain Acceptance

So that is what Pisacano and his colleagues did. It was another major gamble taken in the late 1960s to get family practice legitimized—going all in on making family practice training look as much like how other specialties were trained. As a short-term strategy, it made sense. If the new specialty wanted the blessing of organized medicine, family practice had to conform to how other medical specialties created their members and legitimized themselves. At a big picture level, this conformity included establishing multi-year residency training programs based in academic medical centers, a formal specialty board accepted by the profession's Council of Specialty Medical Societies, rigorous certification exams, and a defined scope of practice. In short, family practice would have to include the same hoops and hurdles other medical specialties contained. The influential Millis Report, sponsored by the American Medical Association, gave cover to pursuing this strategy.

> Fifth, the level of training should be on a par with that of other specialties. A two-year graduate program is insufficient. It follows that there should be a specialty board, certification examinations, and diplomate status for physicians highly qualified in comprehensive care. In terms of responsibility, length of training, and position in the medical hierarchy, the examinations, privileges, and accouterments of specialization are indicated. A new board might be established to certify primary care physicians. . . . The result of these educational changes should be a growing corps of physicians who qualitatively are the peers of their classmates who chose surgery or some other specialty. (Millis 1966, pp. 53–54)

For many early movement leaders, this part of the strategy was not a risk but an imperative. To them, there simply was no other choice. They saw the essential strategic mistake of general practice, repeated from the 1940s through the 1960s, as one of never seeking seriously to embrace those structural features that would have legitimized it better and given it a chance to compete against the new, exciting specialties of American medicine. General practice never seriously tried to create three-year residency training programs. It never supported a formal certification board for its members. For family medicine to have a chance, Pisacano believed that this mistake could not be repeated.

> In short, talking, writing and discussing have been healthy and informative. For this we are grateful, but we are reaching the point when it is about to become a charivari. It is now time for action, not more lip homage. We must set into motion plans to produce training disciplines in family practice, programs that will spawn well-trained, well-motivated specialists in family practice. (Pisacano 1964, p. 177)

As described earlier, by the late 1960s, most existing GP training experiences were still unstructured, remained in non-academic care delivery settings, and involved GP trainees simply rotating through different services in the hospital, on an ad hoc basis, to gain experience. There were few uniform standards enforced across these different training programs. It was a system that produced too many subpar doctors.

> Some of the older generation of physicians have kept up with the scientific developments in medicine, but many have not. This is particularly true among general practitioners, as the widely quoted study of medical practice in North Carolina revealed. This study, jointly conducted by the Rockefeller Foundation and the University of North Carolina, found about 15 percent of a group of general practitioners to be uniformly poor in the quality of medicine they practiced, 25 percent to be only a little better, 30 percent to be reasonably satisfactory, 20 percent to be quite good, and 10 percent to be outstanding. Many of the faults found, such as inadequate examination and history taking, were of a rudimentary character. . . . The North Carolina study demonstrates a real need for upgrading medical practice in those areas in which the public is not receiving the quality of medical care to which it is entitled. (Millis 1966, pp. 3–4)

In a societal age where specialization in all walks of life was preferable, a generalist physician, and worse, a poorly trained one, had no chance.

> Prestige accrues to the specialist; and the more refined the degree of specialization, seemingly the more formidable the prestige of the specialist. Family practice has been left behind in the triumphant march of scientific development which has produced a score of major clinical specialties, some of them orbited by swarms of sub—and sub-sub—specialties. (Family Health Foundation of America 1969, p. 8)

More troubling were the concerns about training and competence put forth by GPs themselves. As Hiram Curry, a GP and intellectual leader in the early family medicine movement, lamented years later, many GPs did not believe in themselves as "real" physicians:

> I believed most general practitioners were inadequately trained physicians. I have thought about this many times over the years; I believe

I was correct. I was an inadequate physician for my responsibilities in Jasper, Florida. Later between 1963 and 1970, I served as a consultant for many general practitioners. That experience reinforces this opinion. . . . . My self-image as a general practitioner was poor, and that of most of the general practitioners I knew was poor. I believed that there had to be professional pride if there was to be professional happiness. Pride in being a professional ordinarily issues from recognition by colleagues and those you serve that you are a professional. I believed then, and I continue to believe, that Family Medicine must be a genuine specialty, and family physicians must be specialists, if Family Medicine is to survive in America. (American Academy of Family Physicians 1999)

Curry's quote is fascinating in its brutal honesty. The Millis Report and other influential writings supported this idea of imitation and helped set the stage for people like Pisacano to push forward with it. If family doctors were going to gain support, the argument went, they had to be legitimate in the eyes of these other specialties and the thousands of young medical students each year who had many options from which to choose. The quickest way to look legitimate was to copy everyone else.

Things moved quickly in the late 1960s to this end. As recently as 1965, delegates of the American Academy of General Practice (AAGP) had voted down the idea of a certification board. But by 1966, the Liaison Committee for Specialty Boards (LCSB) of the American Medical Association received a preliminary application for such a board from no less than the AAGP. In 1969, the LCSB gave final approval to the new American Board of Family Practice, which would have five of its fifteen board directors come from the following specialties: general surgery, obstetrics and gynecology, pediatrics, psychiatry, and internal medicine—making it co-optation at its best. At the same time, the first family medicine residency programs were identified, with fifteen original programs, one of which was Nick Pisacano's program at the University of Kentucky, blossoming nationally into eighty-seven approved family practice residencies by the end of 1971 with over five hundred family doctors training in these programs (American Academy of Family Physicians 1971).

These numbers would grow rapidly during the 1970s, resulting in over three hundred approved family practice residencies and 4,681 family practice residents by 1976 (American Academy of Family Physicians 1976). Family practice residencies would be based in academic medical centers and hospital settings, the very places where other specialty residency programs could be found, which added to the imitation flavor. There would also be the establishment of departments of family practice in most of these settings to run these residency programs. This would create the perception that family practice was as integral to the functioning of a hospital or health system as any other clinical department.

The new specialty of family practice also created a board certification exam that all new graduates, as well as existing general practitioners, had to take and pass every seventh year of practice if they wished to be called *family physicians*. This recertification process was a first for any medical specialty. Another organization, the Society of Teachers in Family Medicine, designed to support and advance the intellectual content of the field, was formed in 1970. By the early 1970s, the field of family practice looked great on paper. It appeared to have all the trappings of any other medical specialty with respect to turning out its own. With the recertification requirement, it looked even stronger in its training requirements. To Pisacano, this was all the better to convince medical students to choose family practice. Still, despite this imitation approach, he retained a healthy cynicism toward the medical establishment. He even took a swing at them while he was using their training blueprint for his new specialty.

My first generalization, then, is (1) that medical schools have contributed little toward the practice of medicine; (2) that, in fact, medical educators have very little understanding of what comprehensive medicine truly is; (3) that the rise of the newest approved specialty, family practice, after many abortive attempts at approval, owes little to medical educators for its eventual success in attaining approval on Feb. 8, 1969; and (4) that, even in the light of this recent surge of interest in family practice, many deans and/or their faculties would not yet be anticipating residencies in family practice were it not for legislative fiats . . . or for the fact that it appears there is on the horizon the dean's delight, i.e. large federal grants. (Pisacano 1970, p. 432)

But the blueprint of imitation family practice followed was flawed. That blueprint conveyed the notion that family practice was committed to training its future doctors in ways not well aligned with, by its own definition, what it was they wanted these doctors to become, which were not clinical researchers, proceduralists, technicians, or full-time hospital physicians. Doing the vast majority of family practice training in the hospital would certainly expose young family doctors to the world of complex medicine they were supposed to help patients manage. But these residents would not be encouraged or allowed to do this complex work once in full-time practice. They would be learning how to do and understand procedures which, once in practice, most of them would rarely do, especially as time went on.

By sealing off most community-based, outpatient primary care doctors from this new training structure, which was based in academic medical centers and hospitals, these same young family doctors would get much less experience doing longitudinal outpatient primary care in community-based private practices. They would not really be learning how to become generalists. It was in these non-hospital settings where they could watch older mentors establish and maintain close relationships with their patients, do prevention and community advocacy, and be the manager of their patients' total-care needs. In short, where they could see and learn the job Pisacano and others wanted them to do by the definition put forth.

This meant that not only would they not get the right amount of early experience and training for key parts of the family practice role, but they would train for the role without seeing all of the pros and cons of what that role required them to do. They would be isolated from those mentors who were out in the community managing their own busy family practices. This training model would alienate these potential mentors, who did not have the time to interact with family practice residents meaningfully in hospitals and who saw residency programs tied to hospital settings as giving family medicine residents only a small portion of the skills needed to go into the community, begin or join a practice, build a patient panel, and practice outpatient medicine full-time.

This reality would leave some family doctors in the dark about how to fulfill the role appropriately. The learning curve would be steeper for a young family doctor who felt more comfortable with hospital medicine than outpatient generalist medicine by the end of their three-year training experience. Ironically, in 1970 Pisacano understood the need for family practice residents to have this type of real-world family practice training exposure, even as he led the charge to put in place a residency program model for the field that was heavily hospital-focused and that relied on faculty who worked there, not out in the community and in their own primary care practices.

> One further grievance: I contend that one of the most serious mistakes of medical educator-administrators has been the recent trend toward the use of full-time faculty in clinical areas and the spurning of practicing physicians in the intimate teaching of medical students. It is obvious to me, now, that one of the major problems is that faculties, in general, have little sensitivity to medicine as it is practiced in the real world. I believe it is high time that there should be increasing use of practicing physicians in the active teaching of medical students in clinical medicine, and by this I do not mean a token gesture, but real, live practitioners giving a fair piece of their time to teaching medical students. (Pisacano 1970, p. 432)

The inconsistencies associated with how family practice training was being institutionalized in the early 1970s seemed less relevant to Pisacano and the field. And at the time, it did not seem to matter. Departments of family practice grew, family practice residency programs grew, money flowed in from the government to grow the specialty, and the number of family doctors exploded. The American Board of Family Medicine, overseeing the training apparatus, entrenched and got the authority to license all family doctors in the United States. The American Academy of General Practice finally agreed to change its name to the American Academy of Family Practice in 1970. There was a burst of interest from medical students to join this fledgling specialty.

By the early 1970s, everything seemed to be working out well. Soon enough, however, as the family practice movement began to stall out in the late 1970s, a collective angst would set in among family doctors and the leaders among them, including the die-hard Nick Pisacano. It's an angst that continues to this day, as the public, insurers, and other doctors have still not grasped the full value of a family doctor; as medical students continue to turn away from choosing this career; as reimbursement for primary care remains inadequate; and as the downsides of the field's short-term strategies have become more apparent.

I have always had a deep professional, as well as personal love and admiration for you. Most people would have given up on me during those long, trying years that I have dealt with the great loss of my dear husband. The perseverance, confidence, patience, and kindness you exemplified in dealing with me will always be remembered in my conscious self as well as my family. You have always "had time" for me. . . .

Much love,

Gladys B.

Patient letter to Dr. Rutland upon his retirement, 1997 (Rutland Papers, Center for the History of Family Medicine)

six

The Struggle to Be a True Believer as a Family Doctor

ONE IMPORTANT THING the specialty of family practice has been effective at doing over five decades is using the image of the comprehensive family doctor as a marketing pitch to draw in medical students and young physicians who think like the altruists we met in chapter three. Compared to other medical specialties, it has always had a large number self-select into it who convince themselves that family practice is the right way to be a physician, and a great career choice for helping society—even more so if they become the kind of comprehensive family doctor Nicholas Pisacano wanted them to become.

These true believers have given family practice hope. They have been the frontline foot soldiers seeking to spread the comprehensive doctor mantra. Many have owned practices. Many have stayed in the same community seeing the same patients for years, like Dr. Richard Rutland. They face challenges now. Their army has been battered and whittled down in numbers as the surrounding health care system grows hostile to their interests and as more young family doctors question what it is they are supposed to be doing. The job of a family medicine true believer is getting harder. Yet, as these true believers go, so goes the specialty's vision of itself as something truly unique in medicine, something that can transform how we all think about and receive health care, and something that can establish primary care, prevention, and community health as the central features of this thinking.

Orrin is a family medicine true believer. He has been one throughout his decades-long career. He is in his late fifties, not old for anyone in the working world, especially not for a physician. In speaking with him by phone for the first time, he comes across as someone who has been through a lot in his career. He sounds tired. He's worn out from the hard work of trying to remain co-owner of a small, independent practice not yet swallowed up by one of the larger hospital-based corporations looming in his geographic area; worn out from trying to meet all the demands of insurance companies, the government, and his patients; worn out from trying to make ends meet in a reimbursement world where seeing more patients quicker, rather than cultivating good relationships with them slower, determines how much one can get paid as a family doctor. People may think it is easy being a physician and owning a practice—the business comes to you and there is plenty of money to make (isn't there?)—but in our health care system, operating a small family practice business is complicated and expensive. It offers razor-thin profit margins and requires a lot of investment. It involves loads of paperwork and administrative chores.

I would not say Orrin is cynical. There is a sentimental yet cold realism in everything he says, as if he were your older brother out with you in a quiet tavern somewhere explaining how he and his wife of thirty years, who you have known since you were young, have decided to separate—talking you through it like a journalist would, rationalizing it. It sounds sad, nostalgic, and factual all at once. He clearly has run through his own mind the scenario of where he is at right now and where he has been.

Orrin fancies himself as a country doctor of sorts. His four-physician practice, which includes his son Owen, is in a small rural town in western New York. It has been there since the 1980s when he took over from a local general practitioner who was retiring. Orrin has always been a true believer about the role of family doctors and about how they should practice their trade. He has pursued his career in that manner. During our first interview, he speaks of retirement as a real option within the next five years. He is from a health care family, though no physicians. His upbringing in another small western New York town shaped how he pursued medicine and ultimately family medicine:

I grew up in a village called Clifton Springs in the Finger Lakes area here in New York, and it basically is a village that is centered around a hospital and before that a sanitarium and spa. It is a medically centered community. I'm the oldest of three kids. My mom was an RN [registered nurse]—she's passed—and my dad was the head X-ray technician in the hospital the next town over. So I was exposed to medical things all of my growing up years and it just sort of naturally evolved from there that I wanted to look at medicine as a career. From the beginning my vision of what a doctor was, so to speak, was probably the vision of the general practitioner [GP] that I saw when I was sick.

I really wanted to be the village doctor somewhere and that's probably where that all came from, and it kind of stuck with me all the way through. I kind of always had in my head that I wanted to come back to rural upstate New York and practice medicine. So after residency I looked at a few different kinds of situations, mostly solo GP practices for guys that were retiring, and I settled on this practice that I'm still in thirty-three years later where an older GP was looking to retire. He admitted to the hospital both my parents worked at and they spoke highly of him. (Orrin, late-career family doctor)

I like talking to Orrin. There is no nonsense or empty talk in him like there is in some others. He comes across as a bit scared of the future, and also quietly upset about how the existing health care system has gone out of its way to take out small guys like him. He does not come across as someone needing anyone to feel sorry for him though. He is a true believer because he has stayed put in one community for over three decades, ever since he got out of residency. He has had the same patients for years, is friends with many of those patients, and has done a lot of varied and complex work as one of the few local doctors in the area. He performs many of the work roles those early definitions of family practice produced by Pisacano and the Millis Report put forth.

It seems like he has made his surroundings better. He believes in the promise of what a comprehensive family doctor can do in a place like this—relational excellence with patients, focusing on prevention, helping people and families work out their health problems, giving good advice, managing illness cost-effectively, being there when they need someone, and advocating for change in the community that improves people's prospects for healthy lives. He has dedicated his working life to being the kind of doctor the specialty has always wanted, even teaching part-time in a local residency program to produce other family doctors like him. Richard Rutland would be proud.

I live out in the country on a twelve-acre lot, and my house is at one end—it's an old farm house—and the other side is the office that I built around '91—I think five years into my time here. I participated with the Blue Cross Blue Shield product that was here but it didn't mean that they paid much of anything in the office. I mean we really didn't even cover those things [with our insurance reimbursement], office calls and such things. So they paid me their rate for hospital patients. I was delivering babies; I delivered babies for twenty years. They paid me for deliveries, for assisting in surgeries, for office surgeries, but most of what people did was just pay you, and the rate was set so there was a lot less middle man. We didn't need the administrative staff. My wife was my nurse and my secretary and we ran that office by ourselves for a long time. Then I moved to the bigger office a few years later with one of the other GPs in town who I had cross covered with and who was ready to retire. In those days nobody wanted to become a solo practitioner, so the hospital helped me recruit someone to that office as part of my practice.

It was the year my daughter was born which would have been 1994. So we recruited to that office and we became a three-doctor-and-one-nurse practitioner practice in three different offices really [over time], and that kind of just continued ever since as things have evolved. . . . I'm not unsatisfied with the career. And even if it was always the way it is now in terms of the hassles, I would still have chosen to do it. The ever-expanding hassles make a much smaller part of the day rewarding and joyful. It used to be I would say 80 percent of my day was meaningful and rewarding and now it's probably 40 percent, but the richness of that 40 percent is enough to offset the other part. But it's infuriating to be wasting all this time on things that are frustrating and don't help patients and tire me out.

It's just becoming harder and harder for us to remain viable as a private entity, because the way the system has been set up now, it's really been designed to exterminate us despite the fact that we have better results. We are the last essentially privately owned practice in this area; the rest of them are owned by systems. Insurance companies pay them more than they pay us and they pay their doctors more because they can use primary care as loss leaders. It's crazy. We are the only practice in the area that still takes care of our patients in the hospital. As physicians, we are paid well below the average of new family doctors even coming out right now. It's [salaries for him and his partners] been up and down some the last few years but pretty flat, and this year it has been a bigger struggle even. (Orrin)

Orrin clearly believes his brand of family medicine is better as an independent practitioner who has built a loyal group of patients to care for over time. He has been able to make the kinds of choices he believes are crucial to doing successful comprehensive medicine. But like Richard Rutland, it was much easier when the health system around him did not get in his way as much, when he could fulfill his strong motivations to be like Rutland, or Welby, and meet the ideal his specialty laid out for him.

A Chip Off the Old Block: A Son Struggles to Follow His Father

Owen is Orrin's son, and he has followed in his father's footsteps. He is a new partner in his father's practice. Being a partner means he has had to invest money and take a salary cut as he builds his own panel of patients. He is in his early thirties, only a few years removed from his residency. Owen was immersed in the small-town physician experience growing up and watching his dad.

Choosing medicine as a career and choosing family medicine, although I tried to be objective about it, I grew up in a household where my father's a family doctor and a small town community doctor, so that was my experience of medicine as a kid and the impression of what a doctor in a small town is like. It was an interesting and attractive thing certainly as a young boy, and then in the mid-adolescent time frame, I pushed away from that and second guessed some of those thoughts but ultimately settled on that. Choosing family medicine, same kind of story. That was my experience of what medicine was. When somebody said they're a doctor or I envisioned a doctor, it was essentially a family medicine doctor or a general practitioner, which is that you're a person that takes care of patients when they need you.

Admittedly, going into medical school, I thought I wanted to be a surgeon. Surgery was something that was palpable and understandable. There was a problem anatomically that was there, you went in, you cut it out, and it was a solved problem, and before learning family medicine, that was interesting and exciting, and hypertension, and diabetes, and that kind of stuff was boring mostly because it wasn't understood partly. I had to learn more about medicine, the problem solving and the analytical part of it, then it became more of a draw as well. So those were the . . . things that led me to family medicine, . . . the breadth of it and problem solving and my foundation with experience growing up in a household with a family doctor. (Owen, early-career family doctor)

Owen is a true believer in how he has performed his family medicine role up to now—in trying to fulfill the comprehensive physician role for his patients, in his decision to become part of his father's practice and make a difference in his community. But he is a younger true believer, and that carries with it unique burdens compared to his father. Like his dad, Owen comes across as clear-eyed and reasonable. It is clear he is trying to think things through. When I speak with him for the first time, he is concerned about his future. He is taking personal, financial, and professional risks most other family doctors his age choose not to take, risks most family doctors of any age seem not to be taking anymore. He owes a couple hundred thousand dollars for his medical training. In other words, a mortgage for a house he does not have. He is only a few years removed from residency. He earns $120,000 a year, well below the mean salary for a family doctor, because right now he only "eats what he kills" as a newly minted practice partner. During his brief career he has experienced a highly concentrated dose of the things his father has increasingly dealt with in his work—the struggle and uphill battle to be a comprehensive family physician in a small independently owned practice.

All of the numbers my co-residents are getting for salaries compared to what I've gotten on salary here has been notably different and at times left a little bit of a bad taste in my mouth thinking about debt and just life purchases, homes, and that kind of stuff. I'm moderately behind my colleagues elsewhere as far as savings and paying down debt. At the end of the day, is that the most important thing? No. But is it always on my mind? Sure. Had I not had this [buying into his father's practice] as an option, . . . I probably would have ended up in an employed position for a bigger system.

I will say it's an argument and a discussion that I have in my mind. Maybe not every day in great detail, but something I do deal with a lot from a general satisfaction perspective. . . . In the moment, in the room with the patient, it is satisfying. It's enjoyable. I like interacting with patients. I like problem solving, all that kind of stuff. Unfortunately, I think my remembered self, however, is not satisfied, and it's a combination of all the other stuff behind the scenes. On the back side, I have a lot of [patient clinical] notes. I'm writing notes after clinic hours. I'm coming home late. I'm seeing my wife for an hour before she's going to bed. I'm seeing my kid for thirty minutes before she goes to bed. I've got never-ending patient charts [to complete] and paperwork and stuff not medical to do. We're getting monitored by various insurance companies for metrics that are affecting our income. As a private practice, we're paying attention to our overhead, and our cost, and our revenue generation.

Am I making enough to cover my salary? Am I making enough to cover my staff? Am I making enough to keep the lights on at the business? And then there's only four of us in the practice, so I'm on call* essentially 25 percent of the time with various interruptions and being

---

* *Call* is the process by which physicians working together in an office take turns covering the care needs of each other's patients during hours when their office is closed.

tied to the phone, which even if it's not a busy call, the anticipation is sometimes aggravating which makes my demeanor less pleasant. Which isn't always the best for my wife, who doesn't always enjoy it when I'm on call. And so there are a lot of things outside of the clinical room with the patient that are not satisfying, and a lot of times I don't know if this [being a practice owner] is the best choice or decision. There are times I think, "What else, either in medicine or otherwise, could I have done or chosen that would have been more personally satisfying?" And I don't know the answer. What if I was an ER [emergency room] doctor, and when I was done for the day, I was done? There are times I've really and superficially said, "Well, what if I was a hospitalist?" Do hospital work one week on, one week off, again, shifts, things like that. There are times that sounds tempting. (Owen)

For a young doctor in his thirties, married with one toddler and another child on the way, in financial debt, having to not only build up his patient panel but meet his financial responsibilities as a practice partner, it sounds tough. As Owen talks, I can feel his anxiety. Maybe it's not anxiety. Maybe it is more the rational analysis of a smart person who is battling some inner voice telling him to get the hell out of his present situation, do something different career-wise for himself. Regardless, it is clear he has been spending a lot of time in his own head thinking through the possibilities.

I think there are different situations that would probably be more satisfying. . . . My child right now is less than two [years old], so I'm pretty mobile as far as that. I will say on the back side, the vague limitation is the emotional and social ties. I grew up around here, so I have a lot of friends nearby, and then even within the practice. You feel that responsibility and obligation to your patients not to pack up and leave and say, "Sorry, it's not you but it's whatever, the system," and then even more complicated is the tie into the family business. This is my father's practice and you feel obligated to your partners, and business partners, and I don't want to put them out either, not to mention, that's your family.

In some sense, you feel locked in because of that responsibility, so again, to patients, to family, to business, whatever, and again, I go back and forth, because to a lesser extent, the OB [obstetrics] decision [giving up obstetrics work] was the same kind of feeling. What am I giving up? Am I not going to be as much of a doctor? Am I doing my patients a disservice? Are they going to be without care because I'm not available? Are they going to feel like I'm giving up on them, or feel like they're responsible for my leaving, or something like that?

The business is tight and I don't know if we've come to a good conclusion as to why. As my father gets older and transitions, he's cut back a little bit so there's a little bit of a cutback in his revenue stream. I had some lagging in coming up to speed as far as building a panel and a practice. We're close but some months I'm on or over and some months I'm a little bit shy [in terms of making his partner payment]. For the calendar year last year, I was a couple of thousand dollars short of what I needed to cover for my total overhead. The viability of the practice and the financial side of things is tight. There have been months we don't know what we're gonna do, and there have been months fortunately where we've balanced back out [revenue and expense wise], but there have been some ebbs and flows recently that have caused us to reevaluate everything.

Realistically, from the viability perspective of the practice, I think the bigger challenge is longevity of maintaining a physician pool. My father's getting close to retirement age. The other most senior doctor is getting close to retirement age. They're both looking at the two-, to three-, to five-year range to being done, and so we're going to have to recruit physicians to replace them, not to mention, ideally, get two more physicians into the practice because none of us really enjoy being on call every fourth night, and it's gonna be hard to recruit into this kind of environment where it's everything I just told you in the beginning. We had a doctor that trained with us, did some of his medical school rotations here for nine months, and was interested in coming back to the area, and he did, and he was a prospective candidate for working for us, but ultimately he chose to work for one of the hospital employee practices because he got paid more and worked less.

At the end of the day, what I want is to be a doctor. I want to be a good doctor, and I want to have the time with my patients, and I also need to be more efficient with it. But I've actually found that the business side of this, those other struggles, the overhead, the decision making about even staff, and hirings, and all that kind of stuff, has been stressful, and frustrating, and not satisfying, and so honestly, if I could just go to work, do my job, take care of my patients, come home and be with my family, that's allowing me to do what I want to do with less of the other stuff. (Owen)

Orrin gets that his son feels the pressure of being a young, indebted family doctor trying to figure out what the best career path is for himself and his family. But when I ask him about the young family doctor in today's health care system and what they are up against, how it is difficult for them to become comprehensive physicians and business owners if they wish to be, and subsequently how they tend to think about their careers, a lot more carefully than his generation, he has a strong opinion on the matter. Perhaps it is driven in part by how he has made sense of his career and the sacrifices he has made over the years. Perhaps, by not directly experiencing all of Owen's added burdens fully, he cannot fully appreciate the younger family doctor's thinking. Or maybe he sees that they do not have enough opportunity each and every day to see the true rewards of family medicine.

When I talk to my [medical] students, I say, "Try to step back and think of it differently. Try to think of it as work-life integration instead of this line between them." Especially when I'm talking to my rural [medical] students, I say, "If you talk to any of the farmers around here about work-life balance, they wouldn't know what the hell you're talking about." I mean, they're farmers. And their work and their life and their family—it's all part of the same deal. Drawing these lines just adds stress. You move around the map more toward work somedays and more toward family other days.

I don't think they [young family doctors] get enough exposure to the meaningful parts of what they do and I don't know how to change that, and my son gets very frustrated about the work-life balance thing. Partly because he's underpaid compared to his peers elsewhere and partly because he has a different perspective on it. I mean, I spend a Saturday afternoon off at the bedside of a dying patient that I've been taking care of for fifteen years in their house, that's huge. And that's meaningful. Thousands of people in this country sit down once a week to watch a medical show to vicariously live what I get to do every day. You sit down and watch *Grey's Anatomy* for an hour, and I get to go sit by the bedside of somebody that I've been taking care of with tears running down my face. Come on, what more could you want out of life?

We have the students do reflections and we just had our [program] graduation and every single one says, "Wow I didn't realize it could be like this. I didn't realize I could have these feelings." Because this is really not mechanical. I'm in this community and the guy I take care of is also the guy who repairs my car. But I think the thing is we don't expose most of the students to that, and when we do they're kind of canned [experiences]. It's like, "We're all going to go to the free clinic for an afternoon or we're all going to go to a impoverished country in Africa and do a month of medical mission." And it's all wonderful and meaningful, but is it real to them? Because for a lot of them, it's not the folks they're going to be taking care of. Their everyday life is going to be the people they're seeing in their office. Regular folks who are not horribly impoverished or horribly rich and varied . . . in terms of income and education and all of that.

I really am taking care of my neighbors and my peers. The guys that I go to the high school football game with. That's the difference. I hang out with the people I take care of and then some are poor, some are less poor. I have some best friends in town here, and neither one of them are high school graduates. One is a brilliant guy who had a rough growing up and he owns a hardware store–gas station, the kind of gathering spot here in town. It's a town of five hundred or six hundred people, but they're your best friends, the ones you do stuff with here. (Orrin)

It is not just Orrin that thinks this way about what a true believer family doctor identity looks like. Other later-career family doctors who also owned or still own their businesses say the same thing. There is Cliff— early seventies, semiretired, and living in the Adirondack Mountains— who owned a large family practice for decades. He tells me that he personally never compartmentalized his work life from the rest of his life; to him they were inextricably intertwined. He never imagined not being a full-time comprehensive doctor his whole career. Barry, the same age and retired after being a practice owner and comprehensive family doctor for almost his entire working career, expresses the same sentiment. Both of these true believers had long, personally satisfying careers as family doctors and business owners. Hal, in his late sixties, is also still very satisfied owning his own well established practice in upstate New York, and his son Horace has also begun working with him. Like Orrin and Owen, the views, concerns, and potential struggles of the two family members differ somewhat. Hal gets that young family doctors have a harder time of it these days.

> You're absolutely right; it is a struggle. When I look at the students that we graduate from medical schools, no one is going into independent private practice. If they go into primary care, they're either gonna join a hospital or a mega group. Their philosophy is totally different from my philosophy and the older ones who came out. They're interested more in how much time do I get off, what's my schedule, what's my salary, what are the benefits, and just tell me the hours. And I would just guess that 80 percent of those graduates are doing it in a large setting or a hospital-based setting, rather than join independent or rural practice. (Hal, late-career family doctor)

Owen definitely seems to appreciate these positive experiences that family doctors like his father speak of. After all, he grew up in the same community and knows many of the same people as his dad. But not having spent decades immersing himself as a family doctor in that community, he does not yet have the same ingrained personal satisfaction as his father. It is harder for him, compared to his father, to build an independent business now. He has been building patient relationships for only a few years. His dad has been doing it for decades. A lot of that rich tapestry of interactions, friendships, and trust his father Orrin has with his patients is not there yet for Owen. Given the way he and his father have to practice now, it may never be. So Owen relies on a general feeling that he is still pretty lucky to have an opportunity to do the work he does. But unfortunately, it's still an opportunity, not always a reality, for him.

> We have a good job. We have a privileged career. We have good incomes. We have nice houses and those sorts of things, but I don't think we're doing

anybody a service by pretending this is the same glorious, enjoyed thing that it gets portrayed to be, where it's a highly respected position. . . . It's a lot of hard work and the business and the financials are challenging, but I think it's important that that message get out there, not to have somebody play our own pity party, but awareness, I think, is important.

We all who get stuck in these negative moments, we do lose sight of the positives and the good that we do for others, and it's nice when the patient overtly sometimes recognizes [that], gives a thank you, but we have to remember that the personal experience of the patients is a small fraction of what they're going through, and that what is routine for us can be frightening, and challenging, and scary for them. . . . When we forget that or we let our negativities of the other stuff roll into our patient interactions and care, that hurts both experiences, and so it's hard I think for myself to sometimes keep that in mind. There are things that are rewarding about this job. (Owen)

After speaking with each of them for the first time, I come away thinking that if you switched Orrin and Owen around, made Owen the older father and Orrin the younger son, each of them would likely be in the other's exact situation and would be thinking in the same way as the other. They are creatures of their lived experiences. I would expect a young Owen in 1985 to make the same choices back then as a young Orrin did, and I would expect a young Orrin in 2019 to be grappling with his predicament as a young business owner the same way as young Owen is doing now. Context matters, and the contexts in which these two family doctors cut their proverbial teeth at the start of their careers are not at all similar. Richard Rutland had the opportunity and a more supportive environment, as did a younger Orrin. Richard Rutland got paid mostly in cash from people, and he had low overhead because he did not have to comply with all of the quality and paperwork demands Owen's insurers and accrediting agencies thrust upon him. He did not leave medical school owing a mortgage-sized debt without owning a house yet.

Orrin has disappointments about the reality of what his practice may be heading toward in the near future. But he is thankful for having had such a long, robust family medicine career where he was in control and did the work he wanted to do. He seems to have enough of this goodwill built up in him that he can last a while longer in his job with only 40 percent of his day being truly enjoyable. Still, that sounds somewhat disappointing to me. I personally would rather not have our most important professionals happy for only 40 percent of their workday. How does that affect my experience as a patient? Owen is motivated to be a real family doctor. He has put his money where his mouth is, but he has serious doubts. Reasonable doubts. Would you take the risks Owen has taken thus far and not feel buyer's remorse? If he remains a true believer, and an owner, he will have to choose to remain fully immersed in that hostile health care system for a long time. That is a tough pill for a young family doctor to swallow.

Over half of those with whom I spoke were true believers. Who are they anyway? They are the kinds of family doctors who, in more ways than one, not only talk the talk of fulfilling the role of an ideal family doctor, but at one point or another, have also walked the walk, sometimes for a long time. Many do or have done the work of a comprehensive family doctor, which means lots of outpatient medicine, staying in the same place, and developing relationships with the same patients over time. Others own their own business or are in jobs that involve advocacy, training other family doctors, or community health. The true believers are much closer in action and spirit to the family doctor definition that those like Nick Pisacano envisioned when the specialty first began. They are the lead vanguard, the cavalry so to speak, in trying to preserve family medicine as the kind of field these founders wanted.

Even today's true believers face obstacles that can stop them from fulfilling their ideals. Some are now faced with the realities of career compromise, increased ambivalence about what they do, and less control to perform their roles as they see fit. Others face the threats Luke, the mid-career family doctor discussed in chapter three, faced—disappointment, burnout, cynicism. These are fueled by a surrounding work context and health care system no longer friendly to family doctors trying to be modern day Richard Rutlands, or simply a professional that stays true to the generalist doctor ideal. Some are like Orrin and Owen, trying to be their own bosses and run a business at the same time while having to make hard choices about living up to this ideal.

The Family Doctor Who Can't Give His Practice Away

Orrin and Owen are not anomalies. But as they talk to me, I realize they are dinosaurs in the world of primary care. Small business owners in a world of physician-employees who do not own anything. Business owners in a world of health care corporations that swallow up family doctors and who can offer these doctors better workdays, fewer administrative hassles, diverse career opportunities, and better pay—exactly what younger doctors, especially, want more of now. But increasingly, older family doctors want more of that too. It's a world where the need for greater resources and scale to compete looms large.

If they are dinosaurs, then Keith also roams the earth with them as one. He is a true believer, like Orrin and Owen. He was not always one though. He became one early in his career and over years of owning his own business, building patient relationships that have lasted for decades, and helping his community. Like Orrin, he may have always been an altruist at heart, but he chose family practice more as a practical endeavor during a turbulent time in the late 1960s.

> I had applied to the Public Health Service, which was, at the time, a draft dodge, and you couldn't get in as a draft dodge; you could only get in for altruistic reasons. So the turning point in my life: I'm about to leave my internship in Madison and drive to Milwaukee to sign my Navy commission. And I didn't know at the time that Navy officers without a specialization, Navy physicians, would be given to the Marines. I'd found that out later. But my wife says, "Call Public Health Service [PHS] one more time." "All right." I do what she tells me. I called PHS. They said, "Just happens an opening just appeared on our desk." "I'll take it." "It's in a ladies' prison in West Virginia. It's a small town." I said, "Vietnam is full of small towns. I'll take it." And then there was silence on the other end. "Oh, expletive, I've just blown it. My altruism has been seen through" [laughs]. And the voice on the other end of the line said, "At least you're honest."

So I got in the Public Health Service. They sent me to a ladies' prison. I was there—we had a sixteen-bed hospital. The administrator of the hospital wanted to get joint commission accreditation. So he went through all the hoops [to show] that we had committees—same four people, two general doctors and a nurse and the administrator. We held committee meetings and we got joint commission accreditation. We took care of heart attacks. We delivered babies. That was 1969 to '71. We did everything. We did X-rays. The radiologist only came around once a month so we did upper-GI [gastrointestinal] X-rays. Then family medicine was born. There was a good family medicine residency in my hometown in Syracuse. I applied there and I did it. . . . And I've never looked back.

I finished there. I already had my Selective Service behind me. Colleague of mine graduated, went in the Air Force, and came back. We opened a practice together, in East Syracuse, we practiced [together] about seven or eight years. Then I got involved with the fire department and opened a practice in the town where I live now so I could play fireman with both—for mature and immature reasons. And I've been there since 1980. I've had this partner and that partner. Up until five years ago, it was a three-doctor practice. We were doing well and were having a good time.

I have patients that I have known since 1971. Not all of them. A few came from the residency. Because my residency was in inner Syracuse and I'm in a suburb of Syracuse. I do a little part-time work with the faculty at the local medical college. And there was a introduction to clinical medicine course. You go in there with a dozen students and a couple faculty and talk about the beginning issues of doing histories and physicals and such. And the faculty should bring a patient. I brought one of my patients from the residency that I've known for some thirty-five years. She came and she was interviewed. On the way out I helped her find her car in the parking lot. She tells me what it's been like to be my patient for thirty-five years. That feedback—that's the kind of intimacy you don't get in an emergency room, you don't get in an operating room. Not only am I taking care of her, but she's taking care of me. (Keith, late-career family doctor)

Keith is in his early seventies. He's savvy, sharp as a tack, and a good guy. When I speak with him in person—he's wearing a turtleneck and pressed blazer on a cold January day in New York—he comes across as the grandfather you wished you had. The one that tells it like it is, bluntly, but in a way that makes you laugh. He's full of gallows humor about his situation, but he's also the type of person who can make you feel like everything will end up okay no matter how bad it sounds. He still owns his own physician practice, like he did several decades ago, but he wants to retire.

He has seen it all. He had a few partners over the years; they come and they go. He was bought out by a hospital system in 1997, after which he became a salaried employee for a while. That system cut him loose in 2002 when they found out they could not squeeze enough profit out of him, at least according to him. But it is in line with reality—a lot of hospital systems bought primary care practices in the 1990s, during the era of managed care. Back then there was a feeding frenzy because of some misguided sense that the local family doctor would help hospitals pad their revenue through a lot of high-cost procedures, done on those very patients the family doctor could now send their way.

> The hospital purchased us [in 1997] for a modest amount of money. They employed me. They paid me more than I've ever made before or after. At the end of five years, they said, "You're losing money." We parted—they fired me. They divested all of those practices [they bought] and I was one of them they divested. And I like to say they didn't throw me overboard; they left me gently on the shore. So we were able to start up our private practice again. We were losing money at the end of one calendar year and we were making money the next. But at that time, my partner said, "I'm working too hard for too little," and he left the practice and went to the Veterans Administration for ten years, got a pension, and just quit medicine last year altogether. Gave up his license.
>
> My original partner from my first practice before 1980 in East Syracuse—he worked for the hospital that I did, and then instead of him getting the practice back [when the hospital divested of him], he went to work for Blue Shield. And he just retired from Blue Shield, gave up his

license. He's going fishing. So here are some of my peers—the second one is my age; the first one is about ten years younger than me—who are disgruntled enough about medicine to have given it up and have seen it in a very different light. I haven't been able to get inside their heads to figure out how their perspective is different from mine. But at least with one of them, it was very clear to me that he never enjoyed the relationships [with patients]. There's not much left in family medicine if you don't enjoy the relationships. (Keith)

Keith cannot get anyone to take over his practice now. That is his dilemma. Imagine working hard for decades to build something you think is valuable, both for yourself and your patients, and then the outside world essentially tells you that it is not as valuable as you think it is. So here is Keith, a solo physician now surrounded by large, corporately run primary care practices that want to swallow him whole, make him an employee, and take his patients. Like what happened to him in 1997. He says he loves the work of being a real family doctor too much to let that happen at the end of his career. He still clings to a feel-good ending to his story. That ending would involve his decades-old practice remaining intact. He'd like a young family doctor to come along to be mentored by him and then assume stewardship over his patients. Deep down, though, he knows this happy ending will run up against a harsher reality.

If it weren't for my age, I would do this forever, maybe longer. So I'm trying to find a young doctor who might take the practice. I have no perspective about the poor student who comes out with a quarter million in debt. It's a very different world for them. I could retire tomorrow financially, or yesterday, financially. I don't have to make a living at this point. It's certainly an enviable position to be in. I'm working for love and not money. So the deal is for a young doctor who wants to be an entrepreneur to come with or without a colleague, come work with me, and eat what you kill, and when I can't do it anymore, it's yours, for free. But the current mindset is that free is too expensive. I spent thousands of dollars on ads [looking for someone to work in and then assume the practice ownership] in our state association journal, in our national association journal, and all I get is more headhunters wanting to make me an employee. I had two nibbles a couple years ago. A couple emails and then silence. I got ghosted. (Keith)

Keith, Orrin, and Owen are a smaller segment of the true believers I interview. But they make me feel sad in important ways. As a patient, I ask myself what kind of health care system is it that creates such adverse conditions for its most prized and dedicated talent? Does a health care system like that really care about me as a patient? Health care is supposed to be different from other industries. It is an industry delivering the most important services to all of us, often when we are unaware of what is happening, when we are vulnerable and fearful. Yet, talking with these true believers makes me believe that the system now mostly cares about bottom-line results and getting the right paperwork in order. I guess I already know this as a health care expert and researcher. But these doctors force me to confront it plainly.

Second, and less philosophically driven, is the feeling of sadness I get when seeing yet another group of professionals unable to control their fates. We do not need to feel sorry for doctors, who remain at the top of the occupational food chain in America in prestige, autonomy, and income. Nonetheless, we should appreciate how much control is passing from doctor to corporation in American health care. For a long time, the physician who owned their business was a lynchpin of the American health care system. Health care was called "a cottage industry" for good reason (Starr 1982). This type of physician had a lot of autonomy and choice over how to interact and develop relationships with their patients. They made the decisions. Granted, it was not always the best structure for delivering cost-effective, high-quality health care. But there is little good proof that the corporatization of health care over the past several decades has done much better (Gaynor 2018), and it has clearly made the system more transactional and impersonal (Hoff 2017). Losing the true believer family doctor who owns their business means less direct control in the hands of the expert that society, for more than a century, has deemed worthy of making the decisions around how to provide care and treat patients. The expert who is also a human being, like us, and who can empathize as a fellow human with our concerns and needs.

The True Believer as Employee: The Limits on Comprehensive Family Doctoring

Orrin, Owen, and Keith represent critically endangered members of the family practice specialty. There are other family doctors I spoke with that, while not business owners, are still trying to be true believers and comprehensive physicians while working for someone else. It is also not easy for them. They are attempting to place themselves into jobs and organizations that allow them to do outpatient medicine, build longer-term patient relationships, manage patient needs holistically, do a variety of family medicine work, and contribute to their community's betterment by engaging in public health activities, working with disadvantaged populations, and mentoring other doctors.

Maddie is one such family doctor. She is in her mid-thirties and has been out of residency for several years. During our first phone interview, she comes across as intense and thoughtful, another no-nonsense physician with strong views about her craft. She wants to be the comprehensive family physician that Nick Pisacano would want her to be. She talks about the importance of being a clinician but also a change agent in her community, although at times she sounds as if that dual role is something she has only recently come to recognize as vital to being a family doctor.

She was a science nerd, as she called herself, who realized at some point she wanted to put that talent and knowledge to use working directly with patients. She did not start out as an altruist. But she seems to be evolving quickly into one, shaped by her experiences working in rural settings where there are people in real need. She has two small children and a husband who is also a high-level professional. There is a lot going on in her life. They live in upstate New York. Maddie's first job out of residency was practicing in a rural area where she was working directly with another physician, near retirement, who had owned his business for years. She was not able to buy his practice, so he sold it to a larger company. One of the primary care corporations that now exist to do what smaller physician-owned businesses cannot do on their own anymore, all the ugly administrative and financial aspects of running a practice. It's equivalent to a small-time bookmaker needing to pay the local Mafia for protection from other hostile elements in the local environment.

Early on, this arrangement of being the country doctor working in a high-need area for a physician-run corporation worked for her. She could make an honest effort to be the kind of family doctor she wanted and build the patient relationships in which she believed. She did comprehensive family medicine work that included things like house calls, prenatal care, and delivering babies. But it began to go south for her as time went on, and she made the decision to leave for another organization elsewhere in the state.

It's very difficult to run a community-driven rural family practice within an organization [the physician-run corporation] that has financial bottom lines that are the number one, two, and three top priorities. There were definitely successes and things to be proud of, and the community up there [where her practice was] is amazing. I feel like we're on a verge of a revolution within medical care and I want to be on the side of it. I want to kind of throw my weight into the side I want to win, which is more of a patient-centered approach to things. I certainly would have hoped that I had the option to stay in the community that I really liked and have been with in some capacity for ten years. But I couldn't successfully bring that [kind of] system to them. That's one of the big failures in my career.

Their [the corporation's] concept of having centralized medical facilities and things like that ran counter to what our patients could do. I mean, I'm in a rural area so there's a cap on how many patients I can even hope to have in my panel, even though we were always overflowing [with patients]. And then I do home visits which just completely blows up their [the corporation's] business model, going out of the office and only seeing one person for an extended period of time. I did prenatal care for a while which I only recently gave up. I also gave up delivering babies at the hospital. It was my decision to pull back on that, and it was during a time where I felt like there were a lot of pressures on me to start limiting some of my scope of practice.

At this point I've decided to continue with the full spectrum [of family practice work] but we've had to be creative. I still do home visits, but we developed a telemedicine program with the ambulance volunteers in the community to kind of help me and go out to patients' homes and then bring patients back to me [virtually]. Instead of limiting our scope of practice, we kind of got innovative and creative with it. So that's been the idea for a while. But it also became a point of contention with my current employer. (Maddie, early-career family doctor)

Maddie sounds disappointed during our first interview about having to pick up and leave a community that relies on her, a community where she thought she might stay and have an impact for a long time. You can tell she does not want to think of herself as an employee of some larger corporation that perhaps concerns itself too much with a desire to grow revenue constantly and avoid any expenses deemed unnecessary, even if she, as the doctor, deems them necessary.

Before this other opportunity came about, I was not satisfied just doing the shift work that I was being asked to do [by her employer]. We dove into community-based projects that were great. But I didn't think that when I was becoming a physician that I was going to have to constantly be navigating and diversifying and making myself more well educated on things and learn more about certain things. Very quickly within the start of my career, I felt like I had to find other options. I became a physician consultant to a health care analytics group and that was interesting. I looked at going toward palliative hospice types of care. (Maddie)

Instead of pursuing these other roles and giving up more of the comprehensive family doctor role, Maddie decided to pick up her family and move to a new rural locale. Working for her new organization, she believes she will have a greater opportunity to be the kind of family doctor she envisions. During that first interview, she is a bit anxious about making that move. When we speak again several months later, after she moved, she sounds happier.

It was a really tough situation, and that's because the corporation that I worked for said, that because I was leaving, they were closing. They didn't actively recruit anybody else in that area even though I gave them nine months' notice to do that. That was a really tough thing because I was very connected with that community, and I feel like I let them down and left them without as many health care options. That was a very difficult situation. I had incredible support from the patients [in her prior practice]. The patients and the families and that community knew that the system that was there was not in line with the type of care we were trying to provide. And they felt that.

I was very upfront with my patients. I spent a lot of time being very careful not to complain, but to illuminate the problems so that they were educated on them. They knew that I spent a lot of my time that I wasn't in that office going out and advocating for improving the health care system. They knew I was very into that [being a public health advocate], and they could see that we weren't getting anywhere and that we had some unfixable problems. When you're close to the community like that, even when it is a physician and patient relationship, they pride themselves on kind of being part of your life, and they certainly were a part of my life. They wanted what was best for me and my kids, which was emotionally difficult to hear, because it would've been easier to just say, "Get out of here, you're no good for us." But they were more like, "You're going to do amazing things, and thank you for helping."

The [way the] corporation [responded to my leaving] was a different standpoint for sure. There was quite a bit of backlash there. . . . I gave them a date, I gave months' notice against a lot of peoples' recommendation. I spent that whole time wondering if they would find somebody else and fire me immediately or whether they would just fire me and shut the office down. Now I feel like I'm able to take my advocacy and channel it in a way that really helps patients [in her new practice] and isn't emotionally draining. It's actually very fulfilling. It's taking time and energy, but without all that negativity. (Maddie)

Other employed true believers with whom I speak share Maddie's desire to not sacrifice the family medicine work role in ways that lead them away from being the generalist or comprehensive physician. These individuals include Ben, a mid-sixties family doctor just starting a new job at a rural physician practice network in upstate New York. Ben has always worked with underserved and disadvantaged patients, delivering a range of services to them. Ben's entire career, including lengthy stints as a teacher of family medicine, has been defined by this comprehensive family doctoring. His daughter Betty is following in his footsteps, working on a Native American reservation and doing it all as a family doctor.

There is Brianna who works as an employee for a large physician network but pursues her everyday duties in a robust way—outpatient care, complex chronic disease management, longitudinal patient relationships, care coordination—all while running the practice in which she works as if she owned it herself and unwilling to accept a lesser version of her family physician role. There is Adam, who we met in chapter three, who is trying to be the go-to primary care doctor in his small town in western New York while getting involved in different aspects of primary care, like sports medicine at the local high school, that embed him further into the community. Given their employee status, Adam's and Brianna's brand of family doctoring is beholden to the larger corporation and its strategic whims. In return, they get some semblance of a pseudo-independent family practice where they can try and function as generalist doctors—building long-term patient relationships, attempting to do different kinds of family medicine work, and linking themselves to their larger communities in order to get their patients needed services. Whether this precarious arrangement can hold for true believers in most instances is an important question, and it will be taken up in a later chapter.

True Believing through Individualized Career Crafting

Lydia and Sally are not like Maddie. They are true believer employees who do not try to do comprehensive family medicine full-time or attempt to fulfill the country doctor role working for someone else, like Maddie or Adam do. Instead, they diversify their work roles in ways that enable them to achieve career sustainability, while at the same time performing other activities that fulfill some features of the family doctor ideal. Lydia is in her mid-forties. She is married and has several children who keep her busy a lot of the time. I interviewed her at the same conference where I interviewed Keith and some others. She is hard to track down, moves around a lot, and is one of those people that make you feel that you are not working hard enough yourself. She is a confident individual who understands the rewards and challenges of being the kind of family physician that fulfills the comprehensive doctor ideal. That was her interest from the earliest point she could remember.

> I went to medical school and I think I knew by my third year that I wanted to practice holistic medicine and try to address everything about a person to address their health. I kind of knew at that point that I wanted to go to Montefiore's residency in social medicine in the Bronx, and that was where I wanted to be trained because they really train you to treat the whole person and how their cultural and their socioeconomic status, and every part of their life, affects their health. I loved it there, and I stayed on as an attending. I taught residents and medical students, and I was kind of a team leader for probably ten years—really involved in the training program, teaching residents. (Lydia, mid-career family doctor)

She taught and practiced outpatient medicine for a while, doing a lot of different things. According to her, it was all good. But during our in-person interview, she went on to talk more about how the everyday grind of being involved in comprehensive family medicine, particularly in health care organizations that worry too much about the bottom line, coupled with her desire to devote meaningful time to her non-work life, forced her to make new career decisions about how best to fulfill her true believer motivation.

> In 2013, I kind of moved my practice a little north. In addition to teaching medicine now, I work in a homeless shelter in the South Bronx, and I'm the medical director of our community outreach organization. I really enjoy that work, and I do street outreach out in vans to people who are living on the street and [I] try to engage with them and bring them into health care. Loving that, when I moved up north, I was part-time with the Institute for Family Health in Kingston, their family practice program, and [I] still continue teaching residents up there. There's so many stressors in trying to practice the way you want to practice, and at the institute, that was really rural medicine. I was practicing in a small little

town [Ellenville] in the southern part of Ulster County, and they really have no access [to care].

They have this little small remote-access hospital, so they really made the family physicians who do the clinic run the hospital, and there was no specialist there, there were no ancillary services. I mean, it was just you and it was like, "I'm not trained for this." I remember being on call one week and this woman had an irregular heart rhythm, and we were trying to get her transferred out but they were like, "Oh, well, an ambulance can't come for another six hours." I was like, "Well, how else can we get her out?" They're like, "We could helicopter her out, but if her vital signs are stable, there's no need to do that." Sure enough, an hour later, her heart stops and we had to code her and bring her back, and finally, at that point, they're like, "Okay, now we can heliport her." I'm like, "No, this is not the type of medicine I wanted to do." I went into family medicine, this is supposed to be happy medicine. This is too stressful for my weekends when I'm supposed to be at soccer tournaments with my kids.

I'm like, "This isn't working, I can't do this anymore." So I left. But what it helped me learn was the opioid epidemic. I kind of started being the addiction medicine specialist in Beacon [after that]. I've been there now for a couple years, and I'm there three days a week and still go down to the city two days a week. I found that has been very helpful for me. I mean, I also started prescribing a lot of treatment for hepatitis C, because obviously, that goes hand-in-hand with substance use, with people using needles and stuff. I do primary care for those clients who have substance-use problems as well, so I still do my kind of breadth of family medicine, but mostly with that vulnerable population, and I still do that with my clients in the Bronx.

When I was in practice at Montefiore as an attending, my patients were so devoted to me. They would wait weeks: "Oh no, I'll wait for Dr. L. No, no. I'll wait." Now, I mean, when I was in Ellenville, they just want to be seen. The Ellenville situation, or the clinic, it's maybe five hundred feet from the hospital, that remote-access hospital I talked about. They would just go to the emergency room because they could be seen quicker than they would be seen in the clinic. They don't care about that continuity there, a lot of them; it's just those urgent care clinics are popping up and are fairly popular because they want that quickness. They don't really care about the relationship anymore. It is a little tricky and that's, I think, with everything. (Lydia)

For Lydia, it is clear that trying to be a generalist doctor in a comprehensive way exacts a toll in time and energy. Things like burnout and career dissatisfaction are real for her, like they are for Luke whom we met earlier. Work-life balance and maintaining it are real for her given her family demands. That's true for thousands of younger millenial doctors, family physicians or otherwise. She resents the patients who think that going to an urgent care center is just as good as going to see her. It sounds as if she has become a little more cynical toward her career over time. She has decided, at least for now, to try and be more niche-oriented in how she acts on her true believer intentions. In part to keep her sanity.

To that end, she has diversified and divvied up her work into smaller segments somewhat independent from each other. She volunteers at a homeless shelter. She does addiction medicine. She has enough different responsibilities now to hedge her bets in case one of her roles becomes too dissatisfying. She is trying to enact a sustainable career at the same time she wants to be the kind of family doctor the specialty relishes. But she is not as all in as Maddie. She is not trying to be the country doctor, embedding herself in her community, getting to know those she lives with as friends and patients, doing comprehensive medicine. She is picking and choosing work roles that make her happy. She is not taking the financial risks like Owen to fulfill the generalist role. She is a true believer in the generalist model of the family doctor. But she is less willing to drive herself over the edge trying to fulfill it.

At the end of our interview, I ask her if she would become a family physician again if given the choice, because I wonder about it.

I think so, I think so. I know you have to address all of the person to really try to help them. I always have known that. But I've always been tempted, right? I'm like, "I should've just been an orthopod [orthopedic surgeon]." It would be so much easier to just focus on that. . . . To some extent, I think that me veering a little bit into mostly doing addiction medicine has been partly that compromise of it does reduce my workload a little bit. I do primary care for some of these patients, but not all. Some of them have their own primary provider and that takes a big load off. I have someone else who's going to make sure you go for that mammogram and you go for the colonoscopy, and I mean, what I'm dealing with can be complicated and has a lot of layers of social and life-stress factors and mental health issues going on, and [it's] hard to kind of address. . . . I'm not the sole determinant of peoples' happiness, and I think keeping that balance [between work and non-work] has helped me not burn out. It's helped me realize I can do what I can, but at the end of the day, I got to get home. At the end of the day, I've got my own family, and at the end of the day, my kids need me as well. So I think I'm able to close it a little bit when I need to and that's helped me, I think, not burn out. (Lydia)

Sally is a few years younger than Lydia. She comes across as very sure of the kind of family doctor she wants to be each and every day. Self-confident and poised, I interviewed her in person at the same conference. Her high energy level came across immediately as we talked. She has done a lot in terms of taking on challenging work roles, working with disadvantaged populations, and acting on her true believer mentality. By the end of medical school, she was the clinical chair of a local free health clinic. She helped implement an electronic health record during her family medicine residency at that clinic. She has worked extensively advocating for and providing care to the homeless. She has immersed herself in the information technology (IT) component of her work, assuming leadership positions in the IT area during her young career, trying to cultivate a better electronic health record design for physicians to use. She has been a leader in her local and state professional organizations. She teaches students and residents on a regular basis. She is a true believer family doctor who wants to engage in work that she believes is important and exciting, like Lydia and even Maddie. But she also likes to do different things in her true believer role, and she wants to maintain a degree of personal control over her career that can keep her satisfied.

I've been at the same clinic in the South Bronx the whole time. I take care of whole families, grandkids, great-grandkids, cousins. . . . I love it. I have real continuity of care with my patients. Then I also do the free clinic, where we're really bringing people into the health care system who wouldn't have otherwise connected, and I'm supervising all of the students who do that. I'm working with several hundred students every year. Every year there's a new board of like thirty students to forty students that are brand new, that I reorient it every year. Then I'm doing all of my IT work in the other half of my time. And then all of my other [professional organization] stuff; that's the advocacy work that balances the whole picture.

I think if I didn't do any part of it, I might feel kind of disheartened. I love the successes that you can have with an individual patient in the clinical exam room. I really hate that our social structure and our racism and xenophobia and all of those things have created a horrible situation for so much of the community that I serve. I can do advocacy work to really address that. I hate that my patients are maybe not getting the highest standard of care, but I can actually create a system in our electronic medical record that helps make sure that people who are poor and underserved actually are getting a higher level of care, because the [electronic health record] system is helping providers give that right care and making it easier.

Where I am in my organization, I'm positioning myself to be one of the people who helps run our organization as we move forward. I've been with the same organization for about twenty years. I don't think where we are is perfect. I think that there's still a lot of work to be done, but . . . I really love our values, I really love that it aligns with what I care about in caring for the underserved and standing up against prejudice and discrimination, which are rampant in our health care system. And that my organization has a commitment to that, and I think I can keep helping them do a better job at trying to live that mission. (Sally, mid-career family doctor)

Several other true believer family physicians who are also employees have followed similar paths as Lydia and Sally. They have sought out leadership or non-clinical positions in their organizations for the purposes of diversifying their career prospects, feeling greater career control and happiness, and getting involved in bigger-picture family medicine work. In these instances, such individuals do not enact their family medicine roles in the manner Richard Rutland, Orrin or Owen, or even Maddie does. Instead, they reduce their patient care schedules and replace the available time with varied work related to advocacy, oversight of students and residents, volunteer work, and non-clinical work that impacts the patient care environment. They are true believers, but on their own terms. None of them look exactly alike.

All the other work Lydia and Sally describe sounds noble and important. It fits with the notion of a family doctor as a change agent in the community, which is what the founding intellectuals of the family medicine movement wanted. But what those founders wanted most of all was family doctors who practiced one-to-one direct patient care, for years in the same place, and in a comprehensive way. It is difficult to gauge how dedicated these true believers were to being full-time practicing clinicians who would interact with and be available to the same patients over a long period of time and do more of the mundane tasks of the comprehensive family doctor. Most are seeking out new opportunities for themselves by creating career trajectories that, while exposing them to work that achieves meaningful social justice goals that improve the public's health, steer them away from serving as comprehensive clinicians.

This all raises some important questions. Do these pursuits by some family doctors help or hinder the specialty's control over the primary care medicine domain? Does it clarify or confuse the public's perception of who family doctors are, and who they should be for them as patients? Does it enrich or further balkanize the specialty's identity in ways that affect how it thinks and acts as a collective? If these questions derive from understanding some of the family medicine true believers and how they enact their careers, they are even more pertinent to ask of the realists working in family practice. These individuals are the focus of the next chapter.

Dear Dr. Rutland,

Thank you so much for the many years you worked trying to keep this body together while I worked trying to destroy it. . . .

    With love,

    Omega R.

    Patient letter to Dr. Rutland upon his retirement, 1997 (Rutland Papers, Center for the History of Family Medicine)

SEVEN

The Realists

Family Doctors Charting Their Own Course

JOANNA IS A REALIST. When I interviewed her, she was a third-year resident working in Boston for a hospital that also functions as a safety net provider for disadvantaged populations. It's a tough place to be a comprehensive family doctor. She is in her early thirties, a bit older than most family physicians starting out. As a Black physician, she has faced additional challenges in fulfilling her dream of being in medicine. It has not been an easy road. She felt doubted at times, yet she beat the odds against her. Her attitude reflects someone battle-hardened from a life of overcoming stereotypes and obstacles.

> All I ever wanted to do was be just like a regular doc, but I didn't come from money. Nobody in my family is a professional, and I get it. I don't know that anybody ever made me feel like I could [become a doctor]. I kept hearing statistics about how everything was against me, but nobody put me in a position to overcome those statistics. You know, every single time I kept saying, "I'm going to medical school," people would always ask, "Oh, you're gonna be a nurse?" And I'm like, "No, I'm going to medical school. I'm in medical school"—like my feeling is something far different than what you seem to think I'm capable of. (Joanna, early-career family doctor)

When I looked her up a year after we talked, I found out that she was a first-year practicing family physician working in another large East Coast city as a full-time employee of a large hospital system. It's one of those corporate clinical jobs many younger family doctors now embrace, where the family doctors are employees, do shift work, and may not always know their patients well. She works in one of the system's primary care clinics, one that emphasizes transactional urgent care with new patients as well as more relational primary care with established patients. It was not surprising to find her in this job. When we talked in 2019, when she was still in residency, she was honest about the potential frustrations of doing full-time generalist family medicine in her career, and why she did not want to do it.

> I know what I think I like, what I figured out I like during residency, and so I'm attempting to structure my career long term that will find what I want. I like the thought of continuity. I think that's why I went into this [family medicine], but I don't think the system is set up to support primary care in the way it should [be]. People always tell you it's hard. Nobody tells you it's this hard, like nobody tries to hide it, but they don't tell you explicitly what you can expect, and nobody wants to tell anyone else all of the horrible things.
>
> You know, I would tell them [younger students interested in family medicine] it's gonna be a challenge. I shouldn't say everybody but lots of us think we're going to get in, change things, and motivate people, and you know, change people's lives and do some good. Then you realize you're limited by money and insurance and people's own volition, and you realize you're not that interesting, you're not that special, you're not gonna change somebody. You know, it's kind of defeating. If I knew all that, like absolutely not [would I choose family medicine again]. You go in to do some good, and there's such excitement and enthusiasm, and you have these handcuffs along the way.
>
> They suck. They just flat out suck. You want to help. You want to help this patient, and their diabetes is raging, but really, they just need to afford food. So they're not going to get your medicine. You know, I've bought transportation for several of my patients. I've paid for an Uber from my

phone for them. You realize that people's problems are not their actual problems, you can't fix their major problems, and if I knew I couldn't, if I knew I actually probably couldn't help, I don't know that I would have done it [chosen family medicine]. For all the self-abuse and everything we do to help others, you know, if I was actually making a major difference, I might feel differently, and maybe I will, one day. But for now, I haven't seen anything that tells me I'd be willing to go through all this again.

People are hurting; it's their health that suffers. But their health suffers for reasons like you can't pay their rent for them. And the truth is you're [the patient] stressed and depressed because you're constantly fearful that you're going to be homeless, and yeah, it's a damn—I mean forgive my language—a damn good reason to be depressed. I can't fix the major things, and it's painful, and I think as a clinician, you feel helpless. You feel helpless. I feel like I can't do anything. I can't do anything to actually fix it, and I'll continue to try and make these small advances, but I'm not fixing it, like I'm not fixing the problems. People come in and they're pouring their lives out to you, okay, and you're realizing that it is like yeah, you're so debilitated that you can't bear to leave the house, but you're just terrified every day and paralyzed because you can't pay for rent. You can't feed your kids, you know, good reasons to be down. Even I would be. I know where my next meal is coming from, and I know my roof stays over my head, but their life is a threat every single day. I can't fix that major issue. You're not taking care of your health because you can't take care of the basics that sustain life. It's wild.

I think it makes it really hard, terribly hard, not to get tired with the whole process. Of course, being poorly supported makes it terribly hard not to get just truly burnt out with it. I can only say I try, you know, but I do think we often just compartmentalize. Try to do the best you can with what you have, and know that that was what you were meant to do. Like the truth is I can only be held accountable for what I can actually do. But you want to do more because you realize it's not about what you're doing at all.

I don't think I'm actually interested in that kind of primary care now. It's something I think I might want to retire into once I can't handle the pace of anything else. . . . Part of our residency program blends urgent care with our clinics, and I've really, really started to like urgent care. See a problem, fix a problem. I don't know if I'll miss that part of it, the ongoing management of the same patients, but I think for now I want to do more acute care than anything: specialty care, hospital care, more advanced than just regular, in-clinic primary care. (Joanna)

Urgent care and hospital medicine are two fields of work that should be part of a generalist doctor's workday. But it should only be a small part of it, because only working in the hospital or emergency department with patients you do not know and may never see again is not true family medicine. It is not the full-time outpatient doctor working in the community and having long-term relationships with patients. Joanna expressed a cold hard truth, which as a health care expert and someone who helped manage a family medicine office, I know all too well, even if I am not a family doctor. The truth is that being a generalist physician of the sort envisioned by people like Dr. Nicholas Pisacano is an impossible task these days—especially when you ask family doctors to fill this role for hundreds and sometimes thousands of patients simultaneously over time.

Despite the personal and financial sacrifices they make to become family physicians, the realists do not have a well-thought-out advance plan for how to construct their careers, at least in the beginning. They also lack an experience and understanding of what family medicine is, and when they actually are exposed to it, the realization that it is not what it was advertised to be reshapes how they feel about their craft, and it changes what they are willing to sacrifice for it. Many find they simply do not have the motivation or stomach to work in a hostile health care system as a comprehensive family doctor. After all, the specialty of family medicine initially sold itself on the idealistic notion of what it means to be a "real" family doctor, while also failing to disclose the cold hard, daily realities of a family doctor's work life. When family medicine's appealing marketing façade finally crumbles, younger physicians feel they have been subject to a bait and switch. This makes the realists flinch at enacting the career in the ideal manner, and it tempts them to pursue their career in a much more individualistic, self-interested manner.

Reality Bites: Seeing a Different Family Doctor than the One You Envisioned

Like other family doctors I interview, including some of the true believers we met in the previous chapters, Joanna does not wish to embrace the more expansive comprehensive family doctor role full-time, maybe ever. The problem is you cannot do it part-time. Dr. Richard Rutland teaches us that. So do Orrin and Owen. Just read the definition of the role put forth for the specialty. There is a lot to do, for a lot of different patients. So maybe she will never do it. Instead, at least for now, she will pursue a job that allows her to do a hodgepodge of different clinical work—urgent care, hospital medicine, and perhaps some traditional primary care where, if she is lucky, she can get to know a few of her patients and, over time, manage their care needs. She wants a job that will pay her well and give her good hours, and such a job does not line up well with comprehensive family medicine jobs. I asked her if doing the comprehensive family role full-time, where she might have a couple thousand patients to manage proactively, providing her with more aggravation and workload in her everyday existence, would seem appealing if those patient populations were healthier. She was blunt in her reply.

> I am not interested in doing physicals for people like me: fairly well-off, educated, you know, come to the doctor with this little thing. I'm not interested in taking care of anybody like me. I'm interested in taking care of people that actually need real help; people that actually need you, really need you, like they need you in ways they don't even realize. (Joanna)

There is more that became clear as I spoke with Joanna the realist. She expressed a contradiction, one I hear from other family medicine realists that I interview. It involves their wish to be difference makers in people's lives, to be there for them; at the same time, they also want to earn a high salary, have a life, and be happy. Clearly, the traditional family doctor role cannot accommodate all these things for them.

> When I was talking about it with some of our preceptors, they were hoping to have me do traditional primary care. I think at this time, I don't want to

be unhappy. I choose my own personal happiness over my career. As an MD, somebody's gotta hire me for something at some point. So I don't know that doing something I really don't want to do right now is going to convince me to be somewhere. Even if it narrows my prospects, I think right this second, I'd be okay with that. . . . The ones [family doctors] I see are dedicated to a degree that I do not think I could be. You know, willing to do those things at home, not separate their home life from their work life, willing to get in early or willing to spend more time at the office. I want work to be work, and personal to be personal.

I definitely see people that are brutally burnt out, definitely, but I would say that a lot of the people I see doing it [family medicine] have a dedication to work that seems to exceed their dedication to their personal life. Their identity is their work, and I do not feel similarly. And I think considering that right out of residency you put your personal life on hold for so long, I put my personal life on hold for, let's see, eight, nine, ten, eleven years, if not more, if you count just working briefly, but I put it on hold so long and have not necessarily achieved the things I want to achieve personally. . . . I've already given up plenty to get to a point where I can just practice, and I don't think I'm willing to sacrifice much more.

I hate to speak on anybody else's behalf, so take what I think with a grain of salt, but from our conversations, I think a lot of us [other young family doctors] feel the same. One of the jokes I make is that I literally can't do anything else and make a salary to try and pay off my debt, you know, without going back to school or something like that. Like I'm too old. I actually have to do medicine at this point. I need medicine money to be able to pay off my exorbitant loan. (Joanna)

I then asked Joanna if she has a significant other, someone who could help her think through these difficult career decisions. She was again blunt.

I'm single, and I don't have any children or commitments right now. Residency took that from me. Yeah, it takes everything, just a life suck. . . . [For a partner] the not being available, the not being with the same person over time, all of that. I think for a great many of us it has taken a toll. (Joanna)

Joanna believes that engaging in a traditional family doctor role will make her unhappy. Imagine that, the very things she says she craves in her career—helping those less fortunate, being a difference maker, having good relationships with patients—are the things she also thinks will burn her out if she is forced to pursue them by being a comprehensive family doctor. She says it plainly, with less awareness of the paradox her thinking presents. When I spoke with her, I never felt I could convince her otherwise. Like others, she has a growing resentment of the fact that she has gone into massive financial debt and subjected herself to years of personal sacrifice in lost time and grinding work to achieve something that she feels is now an illusion. She feels hoodwinked and is somewhat pissed off. She is hard-boiled about her prospects, even before her career as a family doctor has begun. To her, the kind of family doctor envisioned by the idealists sounds wonderful on paper. But she lives in the real world.

If you think Joanna is unique, then listen to Serena. Serena was also a third-year family medicine resident when I interviewed her. She is 30 years old and $300,000 in debt. She will be doing a fellowship* in emergency medicine during the year after she graduates residency. Like Joanna, she does not want to be a full-time traditional family doctor. She also sees that role as demanding too much; making her unhappy and burning her out. Her fellowship implies she may end up, at least for a time, working as an emergency physician, a far cry from being a traditional family doctor. Emergency medicine means shift work, that is, working for a few days and then having a few days completely off; going home at a set hour and not worrying about patients you will never see again; and starting each shift fresh with a new batch of patients each time. It does not involve patient management, holistic care, or long-term relationships with patients. Like Joanna and other realists, she also sees herself as a difference maker. But she does not see how a comprehensive family doctor role allows her to make a difference without being miserable.

---

* A fellowship in medicine often involves an additional year of training, beyond the residency period, where a young doctor gains specific work experience in a narrower area of medicine. For example, sports medicine or geriatrics.

It's something that I have struggled with and I have been kind of feeling in some ways, like am I like selling out? Am I compromising like my initial goal or am I disadvantaging a subpopulation of patients who won't be able to have access to a doctor? It's been very illuminating just to realize how hard it is to be a family doctor, to be a primary care doctor. And I'm not even doing it full-time [right now]. I'm juggling working in inpatient medicine, doing administrative chief responsibilities, and it's a lot to have to carry even a small population, especially with the lack of really good support and community health centers not having great case management. My attendings, they're doing like the job of three people. They're the case manager, they're the nurse, making phone calls, giving results, trying to get people to come into the clinic, and you know doing all of the direct clinical care.

It's a lot. It's a lot of work. It feels unsustainable. I think I admire my colleagues and my attendings who somehow give so much of themselves and sacrifice so much of their personal time, like working on the weekends. Many of them, they make phone calls and things at evenings. . . . Part of me resents how much primary care doctors are asked to do, and it just feels like they're very underappreciated, and many of them are very burnt out. They keep pushing through but they're just very burnt out. I have the normal level of burnout after being a resident. I don't want to, especially in the first year, take on the burnout of being a full-time primary care provider. (Serena, third-year family medicine resident)

Like Joanna, Serena sees those more experienced than her have their work lives and identities consumed by the family doctor role. It also makes her feel like there's a bait and switch going on.

I think in order for family medicine to remain a viable career where people stay doing outpatient care, I think things have to change in terms of creating more structures of support for primary providers; that they're doing more of the direct clinical care and doing less of the coordination and case management and paperwork. I think it's a really rude awakening that a lot of residents go through, because when you're a medical student rotating through as a family doctor, you get to go into the exam room and you're spending like ten, fifteen minutes just talking to patients, doing motivational interviewing. Like I have very clear memories of like this one patient that I met on my outpatient rotation, and doing motivational interviewing with her, she was a smoker.

And after our conversation, she was like, "You know I'm on my last pack of cigarettes. I'm just—this is gonna be my last pack," and as a medical student, having those experiences and feeling like you're really touching people's lives and really making genuine human connection, and that's invigorating and exciting, and I don't know that as a student, especially as a young student, we don't necessarily have the maturity to know that this isn't going to be like it is day in and day out, especially because we're not doing all the charting and paperwork that goes with the patient care. So we're writing our one little note, or you know, three little notes for the different people that we saw. We're not realizing just the true load of work that the doctor is actually putting in behind the scenes.

But I think in some ways it's kind of misleading, and it's kind of a false advertisement [for what being a family doctor is like], and then people come into residency and realize just oh, the real hard labor, the non-clinical labor that goes into the position [of being a family doctor], and they feel disillusioned and, for some people, even a little bit deceived. I know I felt a little bit deceived, and I think that kind of makes the non–primary care options in the field a bit more appealing for people. I think family doctors need more support. I think they need to be valued more, and primary care needs to be a stronger focus for the entire nation, and then I think that'll help to keep people in the field. (Serena)

Merriam Webster defines a *realist* as "a person who recognizes what is real or possible in a particular situation; one who accepts and deals with things as they really are." * When it comes to our working lives, we are all realists. We often see the limitations of what we can do in our occupations. We may know deep down that how we wish to fulfill our roles is not aligned with what others expect of us. We come to understand over time that what we thought was the case with our job or employer is not the case. We may come to believe a fast one has been

---

* Available from https://www.merriam-webster.com/dictionary/realist.

pulled over on us—that what we thought we would be allowed to do is not possible, or that what we have sacrificed to get where we are now does not matter. This may make us cynical about our job or career choices. We may use this awareness to act in highly practical and self-interested ways if we can.

But what specifically makes a family doctor a realist? For some like Joanna and Serena, it arises quickly from the fresh battle scars of earning their medical degrees and making the initial decisions to choose a family practice career. These realists often have heavy debt loads. They have spent many years of their young lives trying to be doctors. They find themselves during residency training or their first full-time jobs feeling betrayed and disappointed by the realization that being a family doctor is not like they imagined, that the outside world cares less about the sacrifices they have made to become a family doctor. Joanna and Serena are representative of the younger family medicine realists with whom I spoke—early-career doctors, and in some cases medical students, who believe they have paid significant dues to the profession already. They feel they are owed something.

Family practice training does not show how difficult it is to be a comprehensive family doctor or how trying it is to develop continuous, trusting relationships with patients while taking charge of managing their care over time. This presents an incomplete picture of the family practice specialty to those choosing it. The rewards, challenges, and frustrations of its work unpeel like an onion through residency and the early years of practice. Such an elongated presentation of real family medicine work, if indeed less attractive, shapes the young family doctor in unexpected ways; it affects both their subsequent career decision making and their willingness to perform the role in a full-bodied way. It makes them feel as if the truth about the career was hidden from them. It makes some of them downright resentful.

These younger realists do not have much real-world experience yet. They rely on an emotional gut response to limited observations of older family practice mentors and their own shortened immersions into the world of comprehensive family medicine. Of course, the danger here for the specialty is that such younger realists arrive at quick decisions about the perceived unattractiveness of a traditional family medicine role, decisions which then permanently shape what jobs and careers they choose. Can these young doctors be convinced later to embrace the comprehensive family doctor role? It's hard to imagine. When young family doctors become realists at such early points in their careers, it's much more difficult to convince them that family medicine is a worthwhile pursuit. First impressions form lasting impressions.

Selling Out or Holding On? The Slower Burn of Becoming a Realist

For other family doctors, realism sprouts slowly from the fertile soil of firsthand experience over the course of years. That's the case for realists like Orrin and his son Owen who work as comprehensive family doctors in challenging environments like rural areas and inner cities, and who own their own medical practices but now find that they cannot make ends meet. It's also the case for realists like Keith who has devoted his entire career to building his own primary care practice, but now cannot even give it away. It's the case for all family doctors who have given a lot to the role of comprehensive physician, but who find themselves in impossible situations to perform that role in the future.

I checked back in with Orrin and Owen about six months after I first spoke with them. If you remember, they owned a business in a rural part of western New York State. Owen had taken a pay cut to buy into his father's business and help keep it running. His dad knows nothing else but being a country doctor in a small town, living right next to his business for many years. When I talked with them initially, both were concerned about keeping their business viable. When I spoke with them six months later, I found out they were selling the entire business to a large health care corporation. They would become paid employees of that corporation. Their realism had forced them to make a profound choice.

> All of that [the business problems] was coming to a head when I last talked to you. There were some financial stresses on the practice that I think were present at that time. And we had kind of actually come out

from a little [financial] underwater at that juncture. The call schedule thing persisted. That's still once every four days [each partner takes overnight call], in some variation, and that's become actually progressively harder and wearing on all of us. And the recruitment ability to get another doctor to come into this style of practice and be competitive from a financial aspect [earning his keep] became difficult. We had no real long-term viability. The practice would be able to function as it was, but as doctors retired, it would just transition into nonexistence.

The signage will change. It will be whatever they [the larger health system] choose to call us. So yeah, we'll essentially all be employees now. It's funny that your email came through, because I was thinking the other day that my conversation with you at that time, versus how I feel now, is definitely different. I'm certainly far less frustrated now, and I do personally feel more hopeful. I'm sad, on the one hand, to be giving up the hospital work. Because, many times, I've had either the nurses or the patients express gratitude and relief that it was me or us that was seeing the patient, as opposed to somebody strange, just hospital-only doctors. There is a twinge of guilt in giving it up. I experienced that to some extent when I gave up obstetrics, and the benefits on the back side to me personally [e.g., predictable work hours, more time off] has settled that guilt a little bit. I'm hopeful in the sense of, I know my salary is going to go up substantially, which gives you a different sense of relief. (Owen, early-career family doctor)

What Owen admits is that in return for a better salary, more predictable work hours, and no further risks or hassles as a business owner, he gives up control and narrows his work duties, undermining his potential as a comprehensive doctor. No longer will he see his patients in the hospital when they are sick for example. Because having him see one or two of his patients in the hospital makes no money for the corporation. It is inefficient when they can employ another family doctor or general internist as a full-time hospital doctor to take care of all hospital patients. His patients will slowly become the corporation's patients. Not right away, but it will happen. It seems worth it to him, and necessary.

Some of these things I didn't really anticipate, as far as being a business owner. I really didn't enjoy it. All the staffing issues, and then trying to deal with all the interpersonal stuff among the staff, because you still have to be a leader as the physician. But all these various business decisions and administrative decisions. Like, are we going to buy a computer? Are we going to get a new server? What are we going to do for our purchasers? Are we going to do bonuses? I'm like, "Oh my, God," you have to both try to manage your wanting to be kind and generous with certain things, while also having to be stern and strict because you have to be a leader and also maintain a business. You can't just let money go because the business will hemorrhage. I'll be really glad not having to be making those decisions. Long term, as a practice, we could just basically go on as we were, until we either sold or closed up and went out of business. We weren't in a financial bind right now, where we had to get this done, which gave us some flexibility and some negotiating leverage. Because it wasn't an emergency now, where some other practices are like, "We're underwater, I can't pay my staff, I can't pay myself, we got to get bought out." They're just basically, "Let's get this done, so I can escape."

I'm primarily hopeful. I think that things look better. The people who've been here longer have some trepidation about losing the feel of what has been this practice. And the things that have made it really comfortable and accessible to patients. I think that's a reasonable concern. But I think again, ignoring the fact of where we were heading [financially], without doing this is just putting your head in the sand. I'm hopeful that we'll be able to offload some of these burdensome tasks that have been weighing us down, and we can actually do better at some of the patient care, the patient-centric stuff. Those are my hopes. I'm not going to get called out in the middle of the night to go to hospitals. Theoretically, my call schedule is going to be more flexible. I'll have more time with my family. My in-laws are down in Pennsylvania, and we don't go there often, and this would allow more flexibility for that. (Owen)

Owen's realism is tinged with a heavy dose of relief. When interviewing him the first time, I was never sure that he ever wanted to work as a comprehensive family doctor running his own business. He is young, has a lot of debt, and has two young children. He has watched his friends earn more by committing less to the role, which bothers him. There is perhaps some regret in making this choice. But not enough to outweigh his feeling that there simply was no other choice to be had. His dad Orrin also came across the same way when I spoke with him the second time. His realism was more philosophical, probably because he is later in his career; he could retire tomorrow. He was more concerned about his son's future. Still, there was a wistfulness in his voice.

> That was probably the hardest thing, at least for me and my one other partner, I think, especially to have to accept that was going to be the reality [i.e., the practice would not be able to remain viable]. You get to be 60 and you realize there's a lot of things in this world you don't want to do, but you have to do, and this was one of those things. Once you hit that decision point, you decide to be positive about what you have to do. Life is change, so that was the attitude that at least I took, not that the whole thing wasn't stressful and sad for me. Yeah, you have to do what you have to do.
>
> I think he's [Owen] capable. Number one, he's well trained and practices really good medicine and is going to be a valuable employee. There's a frustration with everything and there's a frustration with having a boss [as an employee] who may have different expectations and goals from yours. But I think when people are really good at what they do, they're in the driver's seat to some extent with their employer. I'm sad about a lot of things 60-year-old guys are sad about, right? This is a practice that I took over from a general practitioner in 1986. . . . He was kind of the standard model country doctor, and that's what I did by myself for years. As other doctors retired in the area, we actually recruited people to build this fairly impressive four-doctor independent practice and held out against all these forces for a long, long time and were able to give people the kind of care that I and my partners thought was best for them, as opposed to some of this metrics-driven care that [health care is] doing now. We kept doing hospital work.
>
> It's sad. It's that 60-year-old guy sad about the good parts of the way things used to be not being that way anymore. That happens to some

extent, but, again, when I started in 1986 every family doc was taking care of their patients in the hospital, so all the primary care docs around here knew each other and talked to each other and shared insights about cases and how to handle difficult things. We never see each other anymore. We go to work in the morning and we go home at night. I see some of the subspecialists. I see hospitalists, but the medical community isn't a collegial medical community anymore. I'm sad about all those things.

Life has changed, and I get it. I'm not overwhelmed by it. Some of it's sort of a nostalgia thing. But some of it's frustration that as things progressed a lot of what was good about the way things used to be done were jettisoned along with some of the things that needed to change. In three to four years, I'll either retire or cut back and reshape my workload. I do a bunch of other things in medicine besides this. I could certainly see myself doing locum tenens [contract] or per diem work, covering other doctors' vacations. That's kind of just spitballing, quick answer. I probably will stay involved in my teaching. That's roughly a 0.2, 0.3 full-time equivalent thing that I have now, and I'll probably keep doing that. I might even expand it.

But he's [Owen] got to find a way to make a go of this in a way that's enjoyable and meaningful, and tolerable; more than tolerable. You want it to be meaningful and rewarding, so that's a little different. I think you're seeing doctors retire earlier because they don't see an endgame. If I were solo, I probably would not have done this [sold the practice]. I would just have worked until I wanted to be done and then let people know. But the fact that I'm not solo, and I've managed to build this four-doctor practice, that makes me feel good. That makes me feel happy that this is going to go on after I'm done, which otherwise it would [not] have been done. You hit a certain age in life and there's a legacy component to what you do. You'd like to leave some legacy. That makes me feel happy I don't have to have a fire sale in three years. (Orrin, late-career family doctor)

Keith whom we also met earlier, the older family doctor who can't give his practice away, is also a realist. But his realism is darker. It is borne out of being burned before. He cannot believe no other family doctor wants to take over his practice. Even for free. When I asked him about Orrin and Owen selling their practice to a big health care corporation, feeling that they had no choice, he gave me another take, a less optimistic one.

> Their [Owen and Orrin's] solution is only a short-term solution because at the end of three years, they are very vulnerable. They only signed three-year employment contracts. They can be let go. Now, they [the health care system] may not want to let them go, but if they do, they're gone. I sold to a hospital in 1997, until they gave it back to me in 2002. Three other family practices were bought at the same time as mine, by the same hospital. For two of those three practices, the contracts were done, and the hospital fired them. I have learned the hard way, in the words of one of my colleagues, "Don't love something that can't love you back." That system [that bought Owen and Orrin's practice] is going to want return on their investment. They're not doing it out of some sort of altruism. So you sell your soul to the devil. And the devil wants to be paid eventually. (Keith, late-career family doctor)

Orrin and Owen have to believe that they will come out of this in a a better situation. Wouldn't you? Otherwise, their choice to sell is even more painful. With the realists especially, it is all about the choices they make. You look at the choices. Joanna and Serena made their choices. Owen and Orrin made theirs. Their choices look very different in some ways. After all, Joanna and Serena are not business owners, Orrin is toward the end of his career, two of them are rural family doctors, and the other two are urban family practitioners. But though different, their choices move all four of these family doctors in the same direction.

Why Does It Have to Be So Difficult? The Realist's Lament

That same direction moves away from the vision of Nick Pisacano and the vision of a comprehensive physician. It moves away from family doctors providing full-spectrum care, that is, doing some procedural work like delivering babies, doing varied diagnostic work, managing a patient's care needs, developing long-term patient relationships, and working with the local community to connect patients to needed services. It moves it toward being a niche specialty—the urgent care physician, the emergency room doctor, the hospitalist. It also leads family doctors to work as salaried employees at the behest of corporations or to work for multiple organizations in different jobs.

This is not good news for the family practice specialty, which has a lot of strategic reasons to keep believing in the notion of a comprehensive and caring physician, the Marcus Welby or Richard Rutland kind, for all patients. These reasons include the financial survival of existing family doctors, attracting more medical students to family medicine, and assuring a meaningful place long term for generalist medicine in the medical profession and health care system. The health care corporations employing family doctors in greater numbers often see family doctors today as means to larger strategic ends. They see them as a way to get some patients into higher-revenue-generating services like surgeries, while keeping other patients out of the office and away from the family doctor altogether in order to comply with financial incentives by insurers to reduce the costs of care. These corporations do not want their family doctors to deliver babies, or see patients in the hospital, or practice complex care delivery. They do not want them to be comprehensive doctors in any way. They want them to provide the highly transactional primary care delivery they promote and refer them elsewhere to earn greater revenue.

The danger is that the family medicine realists play right into the hands of the corporations. They think that being a traditional family doctor is too difficult now. They believe that what the specialty has tried to sell them is not realistic. They see that the kind of family doctor the specialty still tries to sell to the public and other stakeholders, including new medical student recruits, is for the most part a figment of the imagination. They see all that training they have gone through, the seven years of training Nick Pisacano and others pushed onto the specialty to gain it quicker acceptance with the rest of medicine, and some of them wonder if it is worth it, especially since being a generalist family doctor will pay them less and require more personal heartache, in their minds, than doctors in other specialties experience.

When they come to believe all this, whether they are just coming out of residency, or have a few years under their belt, or are savvy veterans still trying to run a business, they consider making proactive choices that move them away from being a comprehensive doctor and, in some cases, from owning a business. That means jobs with less control, jobs with a narrower scope of work, jobs that do not see the patient holistically or encourage relationships, and jobs with less community involvement or advocacy work.

You end up with a family practice specialty filled increasingly with doctors who are further removed from the ideal definition of the role, and who may have less of a personal stake in how primary care looks on the ground for patients. The realists take their family medicine training and early-career sacrifice and end up in jobs and work settings that often create a self-fulfilling prophecy—that the family doctor cannot be the comprehensive physician anymore even if they so desired. Without fully knowing it, the realists may further balkanize the specialty. Yet, their ranks continue to grow, presenting a strategic problem for the future of family medicine.

"Farewell"
We came many times over the years,
There were a lot of complaints and some pain,
You were always there to calm our fears,
You eased all of this, it was your aim.
We came freely, it was a must,
Because we know it was you, we could trust.

> Mr. & Mrs. Donald L.
>
> Patient letter to Dr. Rutland upon his retirement, 1997 (Rutland
> Papers, Center for the History of Medicine)

[EIGHT]

The Bill Comes Due

Family Doctors' Struggle for Relevancy

IF DR. NICHOLAS PISACANO was the hard-boiled northeasterner whose sharp-tongued oration pushed family medicine into existence, Dr. Gayle Stephens was the Southern country boy with the big vocabulary who sought to help us see both its promise and perils. If Pisacano was a general of the movement, Stephens was its philosopher. You needed a Pisacano in the 1960s to have a family practice specialty arise at all, because you needed strategists who understood the kind of war that needed to be fought and who had the guts to fight it. But you wanted a Stephens throughout the ensuing decades to help recruit folks into the specialty—to articulate in seductive prose what it was the specialty and its doctors were supposed to be about and what was standing in their way that could not be ignored. Like Pisacano, Stephens was a realist. He saw the challenges the specialty faced early on. As the movement's strongest voice, he invoked them with a rhetorical style that chastised even as it lamented.

> We have said more than we knew. Amidst the endless fights, games, and debates of the past decade we have heard ourselves speak a new language. We have become so accustomed to the new words that sometimes we

think we know what they mean—words like care, wholeness, person, sensitivity, responsibility, continuity, and comprehensiveness. We have glimpsed a new vision of what medical care can and ought to be—and we have turned toward it, but as every mountain climber knows, the big ones have false summits which must be passed in order to scale the real top. We've all had our clear days when we could see forever, but then the clouds swirled in and obscured the higher elevations. We've had to settle for less than we had hoped for. We hoped for everyone to have access to a personal physician—we've discovered that not everyone wants or can utilize a personal physician properly. We hoped to produce compassionate physicians—we've had to settle for producing less cynical ones. We hoped to teach continuity care but found that there was little time in which to do it. We wanted to educate the patients but found that we ourselves lacked the education to do it. We wanted to integrate the art and the science but seemed always to have to choose one or the other. Perhaps our unfulfilled hopes are less remarkable than that we hoped at all. (Stephens 1982, pp. 64–65)

Stephens was born in the small rural town of Ashburn, Missouri, in 1928.* He came from a God-fearing Methodist family whose father was the local grocer, postmaster, and mayor. It was his father that encouraged him to be a doctor. Stephens's mother had an eighth-grade education. He grew up dabbling in farming on a small plot of land located on a Mississippi River levee that his father rented and then bought to grow crops on. Stephens became a prized pupil of the town, a good student who attended spelling bees and debate contests. His gift for oration was cultivated during his upbringing by his father, who had only two years of high school education and who was sought out by others in the town for his wise counsel and good conversation. Stephens graduated as a general practitioner from medical school in 1950, served in the Army Medical Corps, and went on to private practice in Wichita,

---

* Much of the information on Dr. Stephens's upbringing and early life comes from an oral history with Dr. Stephens conducted in 2010 by Rick Kellerman. Courtesy of the Center for the History of Family Medicine.

Kansas, with another physician for twelve years. He met his wife, Eula Jean, as a teenager and together they had seven children.

Like Pisacano, Stephens thought of himself as a family doctor rather than a general practitioner. In 1967, he began the family practice residency program at Wesley Hospital in Wichita, which would become one of the first fifteen residency programs approved by the Residency Review Committee on Family Practice in 1968. He was 39 years old at the time. From there, he assumed family medicine teaching and director roles at larger Alabama universities. He also served as president of the intellectual arm of the movement, the Society of Teachers of Family Medicine, in the mid-1970s. He tried to take a day off each week, reading theology, philosophy, and psychology. Like Pisacano, he was an avid book collector.

What he did well besides being a good family doctor and teacher of family doctors is write. Over the course of several decades, beginning in the 1960s, Stephens wrote about family practice and family doctors. Many of these pieces were general roadmaps explaining what a family doctor should do, what made them distinct and valuable, and what types of work comprised the role of the new generalist doctor. He expended many pages of prose on this task. In some ways, though, he furthered the problem of a grandiose, all-encompassing definition for the field—one that young family doctors would have a difficult time performing for many reasons.

For example, in 1975, during the halcyon days of family medicine's growth, he reinforced the idea of the family doctor as "a generalist of considerable breadth" (Stephens 1982, p. 17). He introduced the term *patient management* to describe the main role of the family doctor. This term, consistent with similar terms Pisacano and others used to define family practice, would come back to haunt the field and create confusion and angst in the minds of many young family doctors.

> I want to develop and defend the thesis that patient management is the quintessential skill of clinical practice and is the area of knowledge unique to family physicians. Family physicians know their patients, know their patients' families, know their practices, and know themselves. Their role in

the health care process permits them to know these things in a special way that is denied all those who do not fulfill this role. . . . Let it be clear that in speaking of patient management, I mean something considerably more comprehensive than treatment. (Stephens 1975, p. 425)

In this same classic article, which originated from a speech given to the American Medical Association's Section on Family Practice, he went on for several detailed pages explaining what "patient management" was and how to teach and learn it. He listed a series of twelve conditions and complaints in this description that, in his mind, called for the unique and compassionate mindset of a family physician. Like Pisacano's outline of the family doctor role years earlier, it seemed impossible for any single doctor to fulfill, even in an ideal health care system with few paperwork demands, fewer patients, and better reimbursement for services. Like earlier definitions of the family doctor role, it all rested on knowing each patient well, knowing their life and family situations, and being versed in a variety of clinical areas. This meant doctors who stayed put in one geographic area, put in the time to learn about their patients, and who worked hard to gain an extraordinary breadth of clinical knowledge.

Stephens's words over time belie the challenges family doctors have faced over the past several decades. These challenges stem in part from the kind of hostile health system described in chapter two. They include poor reimbursement for family doctors and the undervaluing of family practice work; lower salaries and prestige for family doctors; the dumbing down of primary care delivery through innovations like retail-oriented, fast-food-style care delivery; the narrowing scope of family medicine work; and the increasing tedium, administrative hassles, and heavy workloads of the patient management part of the job. They are the challenges outside of the specialty's and family doctors' control.

But Stephens's words also hint at the self-inflicted wounds the family medicine specialty has suffered in a quest to gain power and acceptance quickly. These wounds were identified earlier in the book, and they include an opaque, wide-ranging, and impossible-to-fulfill role definition the specialty first put forth those many years ago, and the inability to modify or adapt that definition to current realities or to the personal preferences and situations of family doctors. They also include the heavy imitation the field of family practice engaged in to gain legitimacy— copying the training structure of the procedural specialties without understanding how that would undermine its public perception as a unique field of medicine in which its doctors served as comprehensive generalists bringing health care access to all corners of America.

In addition, embedding family medicine training mainly in academic medical centers and hospital settings distanced new recruits from the everyday realities of outpatient medicine and the true complexity (and joy) of the family doctor role. Calling itself a *specialty*, yet carving out an almost fully non-procedural line of work for itself, family medicine made itself look like no other medical specialty on earth. It left itself to be perceived as a specialty of gatekeepers and patient managers— possessing all the thankless work of patient care with less of the immediate gratification of mending a bone or suturing a laceration or delivering a baby. It tried to look like everyone else while at the same time arguing how different its focus and value were—to other specialties, the public, and key stakeholders. It confused everyone in the process, and nobody could tell what exactly the specialty stood for or how it related to medicine as a whole.

Stephens seemed to capture these problems and challenges for the field. He was not quiet about it. Nor was he naïvely optimistic. He saw, at least at the outset, that being a family doctor in the truest sense of the term might not be understood or supported by many and that it might be a difficult job to pull off well, for any person, no matter how committed. He saw the continued resistance by the rest of organized medicine to the fledgling specialty. While he continued to glorify the family doctor role through his writings, he ruminated about its inability to gain the traction he and others wished for from the very beginning. He acknowledged the growth of the specialty in the 1970s but saw storm clouds moving quickly onto the horizon.

> The rebirth of general practice is a unique phenomenon. . . . It is too early to say whether it represents a real turn in the history of medicine or

whether it is merely a deflection in medicine's trajectory that will soon be corrected by the prevailing powers. (Stephens 1981, p. 460)

Rapid Growth and Rapid Stagnation: The Family Practice Brand Grows then Struggles

Family medicine's self-inflicted wounds were still not fully apparent during the 1970s. If one looked at the numbers, the first decade of the specialty's growth would show an impressive success. Each year's annual report from the American Academy of Family Practice conveyed a sense that the sky was the limit, at least from the standpoint of the numbers. Then again, going from almost zero to anything will often look impressive. In 1971, there were already 87 approved family practice residency programs in the United States, up from the original 15 only a few years earlier. These programs were training over 500 family practice residents (American Academy of Family Physicians 1971).

By 1973, those numbers had climbed to 191 approved residency programs and 1,771 residents (American Academy of Family Physicians 1974). By 1976, there were almost 4,700 residents training in approved family practice residency programs (American Academy of Family Physicians 1976). And, by the end of the 1970s, there were 360 residency programs training over 6,500 family practice residents, with over 50,000 family doctors belonging to the American Academy of Family Physicians (Center for the History of Family Medicine 2019).

Why was there so much early growth in family practice? There were several reasons. First, policy makers and legislators for the most part supported the notion that this new breed of doctor could help address both the cost and access problems in American health care. They allocated funding to support the growth of family medicine training and departments of family practice, spending approximately $200 million by 1980 (Ricketts et al. 1986). While they could have spent more, this was a meaningful investment that helped grow the training infrastructure of the field quickly. The rise of departments of family practice across the country helped establish the new specialty as something legitimate and worthy of using a medical degree on.

A second reason for the rapid growth was the pent-up initial demand among young people to go into medicine to become the type of comprehensive doctor put forth in the definition of the field. The appeal of the family doctor role, at least on paper, for some young adults who had come of age during the late 1960s and early 1970s was undeniable. The family doctor image promoted at great lengths in the early 1970s by the popular television show *Marcus Welby, M.D.* also likely helped to convince more young people watching television, as well as their parents, that this career was noble and rewarding. It looked like fun.

All this said, the family medicine specialty never grew to the heights expected for it. For example, the goal of having 25 percent or more of all US medical school graduates choose careers in family medicine never came close. It still has not, though it remains the holy grail for many in the specialty. In the mid-1970s, it was estimated that 12–15 percent of US medical school graduates were choosing family medicine (Willard 1978). That range has remained the same into 2020, standing at 12.6 percent for the 2020 Resident Match (American Academy of Family Physicians 2020a).* Thus, while the numbers of family doctors has increased over time, family medicine has not become significantly more popular as a career choice among US medical school graduates over the past several decades relative to other specialty choices. The percentage of family medicine PGY-1 residency† positions filled with US medical school graduates has also remained around 50 percent over time, with the remainder filled by US doctor of osteopathy graduates and international medical graduates. That said, in the 2020 Resident Match, only 33.2 percent of total family medicine PGY-1 positions were filled by US medical school graduates, making that year's rate extremely low by any prior standard (American Academy of Family Physicians 2020a). In addition, most years several hundred PGY-1 positions in family medicine can go unfilled.

---

*The Resident Match is the annual process by which US medical school graduates and accredited residency programs find one another. It's a mutual ranking system that identifies appropriate residency programs interested in specific graduates who are also interested in those programs.

†*PGY-1* refers to first year resident physicians.

All this said, by 1999 family practice was the second largest specialty in the United States with almost 70,000 family doctors working in the country; 91 percent of them were board certified and 82 percent of them performed direct patient care (American Academy of Family Physicians 2000a). Family doctors generated more patient visits than any other type of doctor. Many people had regular family doctors that they went to for care. People knew who they were, but not exactly what they did. But this overall number of family doctors, while seemingly large, still paled in comparison to the number needed to have accessible primary care for every citizen in America. And when you added up all the specialist doctors together, family doctors still represented a relatively small percentage of all doctors in the United States.

As the new century began, annual growth in the specialty began to flatline, especially after an uptick in the early 1990s due to the hopeful expectations associated with managed care. Managed care, initially thought to be a boon for family doctors, became their bane. It cast a negative light on them as restrictive gatekeepers who were thought to ration care and limit patient access. At the turn of the twenty-first century, the overall numbers of family doctors and family practice residents fell well short of what was needed to meet the access needs for primary care across the United States. Constant reports and predictions about shortages have been produced lamenting this (Association of American Medical Colleges 2020). Ten to fifteen percent of each graduating medical school class was not enough. It undermined the raison d'être for the specialty to begin with, which was the need for a comprehensive physician in every corner of the nation who could care for large groups of familiar patients and work to help improve their local communities in the process.

Nick Pisacano, writing in 1990, lamented the missed opportunity for family practice:

I remember some long evenings of discussion with those few renegade G.P.s who helped get this specialty going. Many of them became weary of the frustrations and dropped out of the movement, but a few of us stayed in there, and from nearly ground zero in 1969 to today, we have over 380 accredited residency training programs with over 7,200 residents currently in training, as well as 37,000 Diplomates actively certified. Yes, we have come a long way. Other specialties are beginning (slowly) to realize our true worth. Yet in spite of our successes, I ween, we should have been further along in 20 years. Why has our growth leveled off at a point that we believe should be merely halfway?

Our primary goal in 1969 was to achieve clinical credibility within the first 10 years of our existence. We have done that; even our enemies concede our trainees are competent physicians. Our secondary goal was to achieve academic credibility within 20 years. This, I believe, is where we have fallen short. . . . I personally am disappointed that in 1989 there is still widespread derision of family practice among the faculties of medical schools across the nation. Why aren't more than 12 percent of medical school graduates going into family practice? . . . Why haven't we achieved the academic credibility we planned by 1989? . . . How long do we sit helplessly observing the deliquescence of primary care while the procedural and more profitable specialties proliferate? How do we get dedicated young people, who aspire to be ministrant while earning a very worthy living, to cast a look our way? How can we bring back medicine to its once held position as a revered profession? Has the 20 year struggle (with more than a modicum of success) reached its climax? . . . The accomplishments of family practice in the last 2 decades must only be a beginning—let's not entrench ourselves into a chronic holding position. (Pisacano 1990, pp. 64–65)

Yet, for the specialty of family medicine it has been a holding position. Yes, there are a lot of family doctors throughout the United States. But the goal of 25 percent of all US medical school graduates picking family practice each year has not been achieved, and likely cannot be without divine intervention. There are a lot of places in the United States with too few family doctors. Stagnation has been the norm since the early 1980s. The specialty does not remain attractive for most medical students. For similar reasons akin to why the realists and pragmatic true believers described in this book come to diversify their family medicine careers, there are thousands of fourth-year medical students each year who see family practice as "a consolation prize" career choice that pales in prestige and reward to other specialty choices (Hoff 2010). So they do not pick it.

The Definitional Problem: A Narrowing Scope of Practice that Leaves Too Much Thankless Work

The narrowing scope of family physician work remains a serious problem undermining the field—keeping the specialty less appealing to medical students and creating career crises for some of those who have already become family doctors. Remember, family medicine was given a definition that was comprehensive from the outset yet steered away from procedural medicine of any meaningful kind. This meant that most family doctors would not engage in this more complex technical work that has remained at the center of medicine's prestige throughout the ensuing decades. It is also work that remains a part of the family doctor's initial training.

A survey of family doctors in 2000 showed that less than 50 percent of them did basic diagnostic procedures in their offices, such as X-rays and flexible sigmoidoscopies. Less than 15 percent of them did mammograms, ultrasound imaging for obstetric cases, colonoscopies, and cardiac stress testing (American Academy of Family Physicians 2000b). These numbers have not improved over time, and some have gotten worse (American Academy of Family Physicians 2020c). Only 22 percent of family doctors in that same 2000 AAFP survey still delivered babies in the hospital, with over 50 percent of those not doing it stating that they had no interest in it (American Academy of Family Physicians 2000b). Few family physicians in the United States deliver babies on a regular basis now. The ones that do cluster in safety net clinics or rural parts of the country where access to specialists is difficult. They do it because there is no one else.

The 2000 AAFP survey also showed 26 percent of family doctors still doing any sort of surgical assisting in hospitals, with half of the group not doing it also stating they had no interest in it. Just over a third performed minor surgery in the hospital; and a bit more than half cared for their patients in intensive care units. Add to this the rapid decline in family doctors who saw their patients in emergency rooms during the 1980s and 1990s, because of the advent of a new emergency medicine specialty, and an equally big drop in the number of family doctors taking care of their hospitalized patients in the 2000s, because of a new hospital medicine specialty that took on that work, and the narrowing scope of a family doctor's work day has gotten worse. Recent studies demonstrate that even when family doctors hope for a wider scope of work upon graduating from residency, they end up restricting their practice over time and are less likely to deliver services such as obstetrics care, inpatient care, and prenatal care (Coutinho et al. 2015). New family doctors have been shown to have their scopes of practice restricted quicker than their older counterparts (Weidner and Chen 2019).

The data on family physician work point to a specialty that made good on its definitional promise not to be proceduralists. As a result, it has seen the kinds of work its doctors do shrink. Yes, outside forces were a big factor in preventing family doctors, even if they wanted to do this procedural work, from doing it. But family practice did not fight hard to hold onto this type of work, work like delivering babies, doing prenatal care, stitching up wounds, doing hospital care for their patients, treating more complex chronic diseases like diabetes, doing preventive procedures like sigmoidoscopies and stress tests, and performing a range of emergency care. It allowed other specialties to claim ownership over it. It defined such work largely out of its existence. And because the overall numbers of family doctors remained inadequate to carry a primary care revolution across the country, and because procedural medicine and its higher reimbursement and appeal with the public continues to reign supreme, what is increasingly left to the typical family physician working in an outpatient office setting is now more focused on the patient management work that Stephens and Pisacano believed was the essence of being a "real" family doctor. They believed the work of patient management, not that of procedural medicine, was the noblest kind, because it focused on the most intrinsically rewarding aspects of being a family doctor—relationship building, holistic medicine, patient advocacy, and keeping people healthy.

Yet, what is thought of as patient management now is the exact work that the realists and pragmatic true believers interviewed for this book increasingly eschew. It is the work they see and experience as joyless, difficult, less autonomous, time consuming, life altering in not-so-kind ways for themselves, thankless, and low paying for what they put into it. It is the work that these days has less to do with having deep patient relationships and more to do with referring patients to specialists and getting insurance and medication authorizations signed. It is the work that has more to do with learning how to do everything for a patient in a fifteen-minute visit. And it is the work that has more to do with complying with patient requests for referrals to other specialists and using electronic health records to collect reams of patient data to show that they, the physicians, are doing a good job. Whether fully true or not, it is the narrowing of the specialty's scope away from almost all meaningful procedural medicine, and the increased time spent on care and patient management work, that is a big problem for family medicine's relevancy as a field. In 2010, Stephens noted:

> In 1975 I used what now seems an infelicitous term—"patient management"—to describe what I thought was the essential and irreducible center of family doctoring. I did not foresee then that the word "manage" and its cognates would be expropriated by the bureaucratic and economic systems for more limited and specific uses, as in managed care, case managers, and practice management. Neither did I anticipate that it would take on paternalistic overtones. (Stephens 2010, p. S10)

The Identity Problem in Family Medicine

One of the last family physicians with whom I spoke during my interviews was Mika. Mika is in her early forties and has several young children. She has taken a long hard road to becoming a family doctor. But her success as a comprehensive family doctor cannot be questioned. She has been doing obstetrics for years. She has been seeing her own patients in the hospital for years. She manages the care of a large group of the same patients she has known for years. She is an advocate for getting better health care to people in the community in which she works. She is also a leader in her local professional association. Mika plies her trade in an inner-city community in upstate New York, working with disadvantaged and various ethnic populations. She also teaches in a family medicine residency program in that same community, a program that takes pride in teaching young family doctors to become comprehensive doctors.

Mika is a true believer who understands the realist perspective. She helped me understand in clear talk about the thankless work of patient management, why many young family doctors shun it, and how important a rich scope of work is to the family doctor identity.

> I think there's a couple of challenges. I think family medicine as a whole is losing its scope [of work], and I think that is going to be incredibly detrimental to the specialty if that happens. For example, I think that a combination of [family medicine] residents coming through are concerned about their loan debt as well as concerned about that balance of taking care of themselves as well as taking care of their patients, and it's leading them to more shift work. And shift work means you either work in an urgent care center, an emergency room, or you work in the hospital as a hospitalist. I certainly see my residents very frustrated with ambulatory medicine issues, prior authorizations [for insurance companies], dealing with insurance companies, dealing with [drug] formularies that change every six months. I think there's a big shift in people coming in and going right into employed positions. Certainly on the national level, we see those percentages very high, particularly with recent graduates.
>
> I think one of the things that a lot of our residents don't quite realize is when you become employed, you lose a lot of autonomy in your scope [of practice], what your scope is gets dictated by your employer. There are a lot of facets of family medicine that I think, when you stop doing them for any period of time, I think obstetrics in particular stands out as one I think about, it's very hard to get back into it. You may feel very comfortable coming out and doing it, but if you don't immediately go into a position where you're delivering babies, within a pretty short period of time you're like, "I don't think I could step back into a delivery room." And people won't want you back in a delivery room anyway.

I look at my interns coming in or even fourth-year medical students that I interview [for our residency program] who are just so excited about maternity care. That's something they want to do. And they always ask, "Does your program have maternity care?" and we have a pretty strong maternity care curriculum. But it's interesting and I don't quite know when it happens. Sometime between intern year and their final year of residency, when they're looking at jobs, they're no longer prioritizing whether they do maternity care. They really don't think they want to do maternity care.

It's like at some point I see fewer and fewer that are interested in it. I have a third-year resident who is at the top of the class. She's one of the best residents we have. She's going to be working around town full-time for a system of physician-owned family practices. I came in on a Thursday morning last week and she's just like . . . and I don't even know what had happened, but she was just having this rant about prior authorizations and all these things that delay patient care, and she tells me she doesn't know if she can do this for the next twenty years. She just doesn't know. I see that more and more. I don't have any good answers for them. The system is freaking broken right now and so it's really hard to reassure her. Because I don't have a good reassurance. I don't know what we're going to do that is going to fix this. And with the hospital systems buying up the small practices and there being fewer and fewer people having their own practice, which you need to have to be able to do more things you want as a family doc, things . . . are just a little dismal right now.

It's very challenging to broaden your scope of work after you've narrowed it. I would rather see medical students coming in and picking family medicine because they're interested and committed to the scope. I mean, the reality is, if we lose our scope then there's no difference between us and being a general internal medicine doc, so then you really could have just done an internal medicine residency. You didn't need to do a family medicine residency. The scope is what makes it family medicine. If you're not seeing kids, and you are not caring for women and doing women's health, you are not doing family medicine. I'm sorry, you're just not.

I don't think a lot of medical systems are looking for full-scope practitioners. They're not looking for full-scope physicians, even though there's lots of good reasons to look for that. So I think for a resident coming out—they're worried about paying their student loans back. They're worried about having the ability to finally settle down and catch up with their peers with regards to family and life and things that they've put on hold for a really long time. I think it can be hard to kind of insist on this full-scope practice when fewer and fewer people are doing that anyways.

I think we're really hitting a crossroads. I think that the fact that family medicine, relatively speaking, is such an incredibly young specialty that we could very easily just kind of fizzle out if we don't find a way to stake out what is unique about our specialty. If we do fail to broaden the scope sufficiently and show that we are the primary care specialty, then we're no different than a general internal medicine doc. And if we're not any different than a general internal medicine doc [i.e., doctors trained to do primary care but not trained as fully in all the aspects of family medicine] then what's the point? You just go meet [a] general internal medicine doctor. (Mika, mid-career family doctor)

Mika hits the nail on the head. If you do not take care of entire families, you are not a comprehensive family doctor. If your scope of practice is not broad enough to include some procedural medicine that patients also see as important, such as delivering babies; or if you do not go and see your patients when they are in the hospital; or if you choose jobs and employers that limit your work scope or steer you into something niche-oriented like hospital medicine, then you are not a comprehensive family doctor. You are not a generalist physician. You are something different. Your identity is something different. How you end up thinking about your career and patients is different.

This is the identity problem for family doctors that arises in large part from the definitional and narrowing-scope-of-work problems. What those like Pisacano and Stephens, and other family medicine leaders, did not fully envision was how enamored the public and insurers would remain with procedural medicine and high-cost specialties or how difficult it would be to convince these external stakeholders to ascribe a high value to the patient management work that the specialty envisioned embodying the definition of comprehensive care—the kinds of work people like Stephens tried to explain in many of his writings over the years.

Now, it can be said that the American health system has always been hostile to the notion of a generalist doctor. It's more hostile than health systems in countries such as the United Kingdom and Canada, which have government-financed care delivery that emphasizes primary care over specialty medicine, in part to keep overall costs low. Certainly, organized medicine in the United States has not turned out to be a friend of family practice. But this is only part of where the blame lies. These are obvious targets. Another part of the blame lies with family practice itself. It has, for the better part of five decades, pitched an identity to medical students and those who become family doctors that is impossible to fulfill in the real world. A daily job that places them squarely in the middle of all that is wrong with US health care.

From its gestation in the mid-1960s, family practice abandoned its claim to the kinds of clinical work patients understood more clearly. It embraced the vaguer yet all-consuming work of *patient management*, using Stephens's term, that these days, and for a long time now, means something unattractive for too many family doctors. The specialty has not tried to alter that original image of the comprehensive doctor who takes control over the system. To this day, specialty-approved definitions given for family medicine remain almost identical to those given through the decades. It has not abandoned the primary focus on a multidimensional set of duties called *patient management*. In its collective mind, to do so would be to admit defeat—a loss of the kind Nick Pisacano, Gayle Stephens, and other influential family medicine leaders over the years would not support. Instead, family practice has continued to double down.

> Despite these semantic ambiguities, something like patient management is at or very near the center of what family physicians know and do. If the centerpiece of surgery is the operation and cutting is its method; if the centerpiece of radiology is the image and looking is its method; the centerpiece of family practice is the durable clinical relationship and listening is its method. Whatever we can do to preserve and enhance this exchange is good. (Stephens 2010, p. S10)

By not wanting to admit this defeat and begin to adapt accordingly, the specialty has backed itself into a corner. It has allowed itself to be continuously battered by external forces that remain hostile to its interests and show little sign of letting up. It has forced its members, family doctors of all ages, to take matters into their own hands—to carve out their own identities rather than buying into a singular one at the specialty level. There is arguably no collective identity within the specialty now, if there ever was one in the past. Many family doctors, like the kind interviewed here, have taken it on themselves to define what it is they should be doing as family doctors and why. They are creating work and career identities for themselves that are meaningful for them individually. But these grassroot identities produce a blurry mosaic for the specialty that undermines the projection of a sharp collective identity to the outside world.

Some of these family doctors, like Orrin and Keith, held out for as long as possible trying to be comprehensive family doctors. Others like Joanna and Serena, and even Owen, have moved quicker and more cynically to adapting in ways that make them unable to fulfill the specialty's ideal role. If family medicine resists learning from these realists, it stands to also lose its smaller, yet motivated, army of true believers, those doctors we met earlier who keep trying to pursue the comprehensive or generalist role. Its true believers will turn into realists soon enough. That is how tenuous it is right now for a specialty built on early guile, a grandiose vision of itself, and the marketing of a single identity that rests on a vaguer and less popular role definition.

Imitation Does Not Flatter: Just What Is Family Medicine Supposed to Look Like?

In one of his most famous lectures, given in 1979 and titled "Family Practice as Counterculture," Stephens chastised the young specialty's continued focus on imitating the rest of organized medicine. He believed this imitation, and the specialty's felt need to be viewed "like the rest of medicine" in terms of adequate rigor and preparation, stifled the growth of the very qualities required for family practice to grow its own unique identity as a "counterculture" movement in medicine—becoming better known to all and enhancing its value as a part of society. He believed that the specialty had gone too far in the direction of conformity. Referring to one of his own beloved organizations, the Society of Teachers of Family Medicine, he wrote:

> Family practice as a part of the medical professional bureaucracy quite clearly began as a sect (though we might not like this term) and has already moved along several lines to become a "church," i.e., to take on the characteristics of the dominant professional organizations. The Society of Teachers of Family Medicine is a particularly suitable organization in which to study this process of transformation. I have read many records of minutes from the Board of Directors meetings with these ideas in mind, and it is uncanny how many of the issues that have consumed hours of debate can be understood by means of this model.
>
> The founders of this Society quite clearly intended to create an organization of committed (i.e., saved) members from any of the health professions who were actively engaged in teaching and propagating family medicine. We were informal, egalitarian, evangelistic, and certainly propertyless. We did not want to become political, and many of us were suspicious of other organizations that might dominate us or dilute our purposes. We were critical of the dominant medical education culture (AAMC, medical school faculties), and we depended upon volunteer or part-time leaders.
>
> Over the years we have tended to become a much more formal organization, accepting a political responsibility to represent our discipline in the medical bureaucracy and struggling for funds. We have imposed restraint on members' participation in meetings; now there are committees who determine who may speak or make presentations, and our activities are increasingly delegated to a paid professional staff. We have evolved an orthodoxy of beliefs and practices by which we judge each other and outsiders. In short, we are fast becoming a church.
>
> I do not present these ideas in a pejorative or derogatory way. I am attempting to describe rather than judge. My purpose is to call attention to our own evolution and to ask whether or not this is what we really

want to do. Is our own best interest to be served by moving as quickly as we can to resemble the rest of the medical bureaucracy, or do we have interests that can best be served by our remaining a sect? We have gotten a lot of mileage out of our minority, sectarian status. Why do we want to abandon it so quickly? I do not expect anyone to answer these questions. They are not the sort that can be answered by appointing another committee, doing another survey, or taking a vote. (Stephens 1979, pp. 105–106)

By the 1980s and 1990s, the specialty of family medicine looked on paper like other clinical specialties. But only on paper—board certification; a three-year residency program; departments of family practice based in academic medical centers and hospitals; full-time teaching faculty responsible for furthering the intellectual rigor of the specialty; and a large, organized professional association, the American Academy of Family Physicians (AAFP), that sought to advance the collective interests of family doctors nationally. Nick Pisacano's push to pitch family medicine as a new specialty, deserving of the same prestige as other established ones, had in many ways been key to the early success and growth of the field.

It had diminishing returns though. As Stephens and others noted over time, the pitch of family medicine as a specialty co-opted it into organized medicine in a way that undermined its ability to take on other specialties when needed, show the public how different it was, and fight for its own unique place in the American health care system. How could you be counterculture if you copied the existing medical culture? The answer is you could not. As a specialty, family medicine exhibited a certain laziness when trying to define what its members could and should be doing. It repeated similar role definitions throughout the decades with little change. It avoided opportunities to hold on to or reacquire important work, such as hospital and emergency medicine, opting instead to cling to the fantasy of the comprehensive family doctor who could do it all and wanted to. It never sought to reinvent itself as needed.

Generalizations about comprehensive medicine, patient management, and other vague work labels ascribed to the field never evolved into greater precision regarding the kinds of clinical activities family doctors could perform on a regular basis, how much these activities should be worth, and what family doctors could do for patients that other types of doctors could not. Remaining a specialty that could only define its work "generally," with long lists of management and coordination activities, created confusion for patients. Patients who could not grasp why a family doctor, if also trained as a specialist, could not or would not do certain types of procedural or more complex medical work, or who could not or would not visit with them in the hospital or emergency room, or who often referred them to other doctors to take care of their needs. In the September 2, 1988, issue of the *Journal of the American Medical Association*, a joint AMA/AAFP council examining the future of family practice stated, with regards to public perceptions of family doctors:

> Beyond the scope of the medical profession, anecdotal information indicates that family physicians are faced with public misconceptions. There does not seem to be a widespread public understanding that family practice is a bona fide specialty. Although more and more patients are interested in having a single physician as the provider of primary care who treats the patient in the context of his or her family, there is a perception that this type of physician no longer exists. (American Medical Association 1988, p. 1275)

In 2002, seven national organizations dedicated to promoting the specialty of family medicine created the Future of Family Medicine project. This project was an attempt to try and turn the increasingly negative situation for the specialty around before it was too late. The stated goal of the project was "to develop a strategy to transform and renew the discipline of family medicine to meet the needs of patients in a changing health care environment" (Future of Family Medicine 2004, p. S3). Much hope was placed on this project and task forces and intellectual firepower were brought to bear on discussing the various problems causing a decline in the field. As part of this project, information was collected from a variety of stakeholders about the perceptions of family doctors. This research concluded:

Family physicians are not well recognized by the public for what they are and what they do. Patients have a hard time differentiating family medicine from other primary care physician specialties, notably not distinguishing clearly between family medicine and general internal medicine. Indeed, the words "family" and "practitioner" were often found to confuse people and suggested to some that family physicians lack scientific background and competence. (Future of Family Medicine 2004, S7)

This lack of public understanding of what family doctors could and should do has impacted how insurers monetize the value of the services they provide. Over the decades, and as we saw in chapter two, many insurers have consistently questioned why they should pay more for activities that the public seems to value less and that are somewhat ill-specified in terms of the time and resources they take to perform.

Of course, part of the dilemma once again returns to the fact that family medicine simultaneously has always sold itself as a specialty like any other—in governance structures, training processes, and intellectual rigor—while also trying to sell the notion that it can provide the generalist doctor on every street corner in America. Early on, the field pitched this message hard. It tried to amplify initial enthusiasm for a new kind of doctor who might fix the cost and access problems in American health care. On its own, that pitch was fine. But pursuing these two paths toward legitimacy at the same time—being a specialty that looked and trained on paper like all the others *yet* having a scope of work that was more general and relational rather than procedural—confused people. It made them ambivalent about family doctors.

After all, specialists, in the strictest sense, were supposed to be doctors that could not do it all, as family doctors claimed they could. Specialists were not supposed to be abundantly available, like family doctors wanted to be. True specialists were costly, high-level technicians who only involved themselves in specific instances of patient malaise. Their supply was carefully controlled by organized medicine and their professional associations to keep a sense among the public and insurers that their scarcity made them valuable and expensive. They were not supposed to be on every street corner of America like family doctors.

Specialists like orthopedists and neurologists did not claim to advocate for patient interests in the community, or advance social justice causes, or care for entire families. They did not ask to manage patients' total-care needs or keep them healthy. They existed to fix something specifically wrong with the patient at a given moment in time. Then send them on their way. That was it.

Family practice was supposed to be different, though, even as a specialty. It was supposed to help change society for the better by helping to improve community health, empower patients through healthy behaviors, and improve the entirety of a patient's well-being—physical, mental, and even spiritual. It was supposed to be everywhere, concerning itself with producing vast armies of doctors who would develop long-term relationships with patients, handle everything and anything that came their way, or at least manage it. The heavy emphasis on making it look like every other specialty in form but not substance undermined that goal. In the end, no one could quite figure out what these doctors were all about, including many of those who were in the specialty itself.

The training also misaligned with the desired role definition. This was yet another problem with the imitation approach. If by definition family doctors were not to be proceduralists; if they would not end up working primarily in hospitals where other specialists clustered; and if they were instead embedded in the local community performing outpatient medicine, advocacy, and family-centered care, then they needed to be trained differently than everyone else. They needed to train and work in those practice settings where they could best gain that experience and begin to get to know their patients long-term. But as noted earlier, most family medicine residency programs were, and still are, closely affiliated with, or housed directly in, academic medical centers, where departments of family practice and their faculty are located. Thus, much family practice training is overseen and done within the corporate orbit of the large medical center itself. To show they are like other residents, trained with the same disciplinary rigor, family medicine residents still receive heavy doses of inpatient medicine, and they still rotate through various procedure-oriented departments of the hospital, learning how to do procedures and technical medicine. For most, the outpatient medicine they learn is often based in some satellite office or clinic of the academic medical center.

Like all residents, family practice residents are the cheap labor that help clinics and practices make ends meet, and they also provide care to underserved and uninsured patient populations (Hurt 2017). But such practice sites provide less opportunity to work longitudinally with entire families, do continuous care, or see the full range of patient management work that the family doctor role embodies (Brown and Irwin 2018). Many patients at these sites come and go. This factor, combined with outpatient medicine rotations that last months rather than years, limits opportunities for the family medicine resident to see the longer-term results of their prevention work or to reap the rewards of having an ongoing relationship with a patient. The outpatient medicine work in family medicine residency programs tends to be fragmented and intermingled with the ongoing specialty and other hospital work these residents must perform.

This reality, still very much the case today, has produced a misalignment between how young family doctors prepare for the realities of what the family medicine specialty ideally wants its new recruits to do once working full-time on their own. It has separated generations of young family doctors from the Dr. Richard Rutland–type family physicians that they could have trained under, working in their practices out in the local community—practices that had stable patient populations, where the doctors knew and treated entire families, and where the opportunities to provide holistic care were greater. The imitation approach denied many young family doctors the opportunity to see, in greater depth, what the upsides and downsides of real family medicine were all about. Too much imitation has led to young family doctors that often do not know how they truly feel about doing outpatient medicine in the community full-time.

In 1980, Stephens once again harped on the problems of imitation and conformity, that is, family medicine's trying to look and think like other specialties at the expense of underselling that which many in the movement had presumed would make it a vital, accepted, and prestigious part of health care. He chided his own colleagues for thinking that the rest of organized medicine would simply allow family medicine to assume a co-equal role. He raised the specter that such an all-encompassing and opaque definition of the family doctor role, realistic or not, had muddled the specialty's identity with the public and others. He felt this created disbelief on the part of some that such a role could be fulfilled by a single type of doctor, given medicine's complexity.

> During the past 15 years general/family practice has experienced a rebirth that in its own way has involved us in conflict with the dominant powers in medicine. . . . The opposition to general/family practice has come mainly from medical schools, hospitals and other specialty organizations. Even though we have secured an academic beachhead within most of the public medical schools, on the whole they are not keen to identify themselves as schools for family doctors, though they cling tenaciously to the myth of the undifferentiated doctor as the typical product of their undergraduate curricula. Hospitals and specialty organizations have been vigilant to see that family doctors are either excluded or severely limited in their access to the high technology of medicine.
>
> The battle for status within medicine has largely had the effect of confusing the general public, and they look on with increasing impatience; by and large, they do not understand what all the fuss is about, why they cannot have both high technology medicine and personal medicine when they need it. Clearly, general/family practice exposes a nerve of great sensitivity in the body politic of medicine. To some it seems retrogressive and anti-intellectual, to others simply impossible; they do not understand how a general practitioner of any type can keep up with the explosion of medical information and they cannot get past the notion that one must be a "super doc"—a feat that is manifestly impossible except for a few geniuses. What now that the rebirth of general/family practice has occurred? Where do we go from here now that we have emerged from a long gestation and can see the light of a new day? (Stephens 1981, p. 460)

Stephens's statement is telling in its brutal honesty. Ironically, it also could have been used in referring to the sentiment and challenges the field of general practice faced twenty years earlier. Perceived as anti-intellectual and unable to keep up with the complexities of medicine? That was once the field of general practice. Spurned by medical schools and kept from the mainstream of hospital and technological medicine? That also was general practice. Over a decade into the establishment and growth of family practice, similar concerns were being expressed about its standing by one of its most thoughtful leaders. These concerns persist to the present day. It puts family practice in an uphill battle for relevance in both organized medicine and with the public.

The Struggle for Relevancy: Family Doctors and the Balkanization of the Specialty

On the ground, and as we have heard from those interviewed in this book, the view of family practice is one of an increasingly balkanized specialty. This is not only validated by the story here. The specialty itself now essentially admits it. A quick look at the American Academy of Family Physicians' Career Options in Family Medicine web page shows several career paths family doctors may pursue full-time, including working as public health professionals, as hospitalists, in emergency rooms, and in urgent care centers (American Academy of Family Physicians 2020b). The web page does not advocate for family doctors to fill all these roles, but instead steers them toward a career doing only one of them full-time. This is an acknowledgment that family doctors may, and do, pursue different career paths. Most of these roles have little to do with what has been defined as *comprehensive family medicine* in this book—a definition that has been spread consistently and over time by the specialty and its leadership, and one that is still vividly present on the AAFP website.

> Family medicine integrates a broad-spectrum approach to primary care with the consideration of health-impacting social determinants and community factors, while also serving as an advocate for the patient in an increasingly complex health care system. Unlike other narrowly focused specialties, family medicine includes the biological, clinical, and behavioral sciences, encompassing all ages, sexes, each organ system, and

every disease entity. The focus of a family physician is the whole person. They shepherd male and female patients of all ages through the complex health system and coordinate the care of their health. By building relationships with their patients over time, family physicians are able to develop a comprehensive understanding of their patients' health and offer insightful, personal guidance and treatment.

The patient-physician relationship is at the heart of family medicine. Beyond reported concerns, family physicians take the time to consider additional health factors in their patients' lives, including family and community situations and relationships. While there are similarities between family medicine and the other primary care specialties, it is the extent to which family physicians value, develop, nurture, and maintain a relationship with each patient that distinguishes family medicine from all other specialties. (American Academy of Family Physicians 2020b)

Most of these other jobs that family doctors perform in hospitals, emergency departments, public health agencies, and urgent care centers do not involve long-term, patient relationship building, whole-person care, or family-focused care. They involve episodic, fragmented, and short-term care, often with unknown patients and for discrete illnesses. Or, as in the case of public health work, they involve no direct patient care at all. Those family doctors performing these jobs know that, and as we have discussed, many take the trade-offs from not doing the comprehensive family doctor role in return for other benefits that accrue to themselves and their careers. It is remarkable that the specialty's professional association can still define family medicine and the role of the family doctor in the same traditional manner and yet also promote careers for family physicians that depart greatly from that definition and role.

Who cares about the balkanization of a medical specialty? Why is it a big deal? Why are issues around the lack of a collective identity and misaligned definitions for family doctors so relevant to understanding the future of this specialty? Should and can a narrowing scope of work be turned around? Can the reality of family doctors choosing their own customized career paths that draw the specialty further away from its traditional roots be stopped? Should it be stopped, and if so, how? This analysis has already answered some of these questions. Others are probably unanswerable, relying more on speculation. Yet they all strike at the heart of whether family practice can survive well into the future in any recognizable form relative to what its founders wanted. Or, instead, if it transforms into something completely different or continues to become less important in health care. A betting person might say it will have to transform into something different to remain important.

Stephens saw it all quite clearly as far back as the late 1970s. Maybe earlier. He saw the problems of a fantastical, unrealistic definition; the problems of trying to be all things to all people; the problems of imitation and conformity; the problems of poor branding to the outside world; and the problems of having a massive inferiority complex as a field of medicine. He saw the error of a field constantly trying to distance itself from its general practitioner past while calling itself a generalist specialty.

> On balance, I judge that we have squandered some public credibility in
> our evolution despite our success in having created a specialty. We probably
> confused the public early on when we changed our name from general
> practice to family practice, and we confused ourselves in drawing finer
> distinctions with the addition of family medicine, community medicine,
> and primary care. We all know the reasons for these name changes, but
> they held no interest for the public, conveyed no weight of meaning, and
> sometimes allowed us to mistake the cart for the horse. In retrospect, our
> preoccupation with defining family medicine as an academic discipline
> was probably excessive. Some of the perceived need to do this was inflicted
> on us politically by other specialty boards whose members controlled
> the club we wished to join—the American Board of Medical Specialties.
> Indeed, William Ruhe, executive director of the AMA's Council of Medical
> Education, who was privy to the negotiations for approval of the American Board of Family Practice, once acknowledged that we were subject to
> greater demands for definition than any other specialty board. But most of
> the pressure was self-inflicted by our earnest desires to become legitimate in
> a way that general practice never was. Our debates about the family as a
> unit of care, the role of behavioral sciences in medical practice, and the

meaning of community medicine led us down some blind alleys that have not stood the test of time.

Ed Pellegrino, a friendly critic, once called us "mutants," meaning that we created a package of services that was more than the public wanted, needed, or understood. The public wanted accessibility to ordinary services at reasonable cost, but we wanted utopia. In some respects, we have recapitulated the dysfunctional phylogeny of mainstream medicine by fragmenting our basic role into niche jobs and subspecialization that subverts continuity and comprehensiveness of medical care. We took a hit to our public credibility when we were suckered into gatekeeping by managed care organizations. We ought to have nurtured our main asset better and demanded from our educational settings the permissions and wherewithal to prepare students and residents for full-service practice in communities of need. (Stephens 2001, pp. 250–251)

Asking the big questions is fine. Yet often those questions remain theoretical and are ignored. It's better to think about actionable items that could be implemented in one form or another. The specialty of family medicine needs to do things differently, and fast. Time's a wastin', as they say. I personally do not know if it is too late to save family practice from the clutches of a corporatized health care system licking its chops at transforming primary care in a manner that serves its own interests. But I do know the hour is getting near, much like it was for general practice in the late 1950s. The last chapter gets into specific strategies that might, with a combination of dumb luck and great execution, help turn things around or at least stave off what seems like the inevitable end.

June 1997

Dear Dr. Rutland,

  . . . Memory doesn't fade, however, when I think of the many occasions
you have been there when the need was very real. Newborn's tractor
accidents and miscarriages stand out vividly in my mind. Thank you,
also for the long, loving care you gave our parents. . . .

  Sincerely,

  Betty F.

  Patient letter to Dr. Rutland upon his retirement, 1997 (Rutland
  Papers, Center for the History of Family Medicine)

NINE

A Top-Ten List for Saving Family Doctors

A CRITIQUE IS ONE THING. Solving problems is another. This chapter provides a small contribution to the latter goal. I do not presume, based on my analysis or expertise in primary care system transformation, to know if and how family practice can be saved. If the thesis of this book conveys anything, it is that family practice is at a tipping point—a point its own Future of Family Medicine (FFM) report, in the early 2000s, said was coming in "15 or 20 years" without significant changes:

> The FFM Project Leadership Committee concluded that unless there are changes in the broader health care system and within the specialty, the position of family medicine in the United States may be untenable in a 10- to 20-year time frame, which would be detrimental to the health of the American public. (Future of Family Medicine Project Leadership Committee 2004, S8)

That is not me talking. It is the officially sanctioned committee organized twenty years ago by the American Academy of Family Physicians to help save family medicine. Is the position of family medicine in the United States untenable now? Perhaps. But the changes called for in the landmark FFM report did not go nearly far enough. They were inside-the-box ideas that did not get at the strategic problems noted in this book or at the evolving everyday realities of the specialty or its doctors. They assumed a status quo with respect to the specialty and suggested general and uninspired improvements—as if the decades-long problems of identity, brand, definition, imitation, and work scope outlined in this book did not exist; as if family doctors were not already, in the year 2000, focusing on constructing their own sustainable career paths. There were recommendations about giving family doctors "lifelong learning," "implementing" electronic health records, "enhancing" family medicine education, "enhancing" the science of family medicine, and "improving" quality of care (Future of Family Medicine Project Leadership Committee 2004). But they are purely tactical suggestions ignoring most of the strategic challenges facing family medicine above.

It's not good enough, as the subsequent years have proved. The cold hard reality now is that many patients seem oblivious to the potential value of having a family doctor; they have no problem increasingly getting their primary care from a variety of fast-food-style service outlets that deliver cheaper and quicker but less comprehensive and personal primary care; and they still do not have a good understanding of what it is these doctors do (Hoff 2017). Insurers remain permanently ambivalent about adequately funding primary care services. The increased focus on value-based health care, while seemingly advantageous for family doctors because it might give them more control, presents numerous additional administrative costs and workload issues for these physicians. Ones they do not like. They do not stand to make more money from this new payment system. But they will work harder and get hassled more.

We have covered the key contextual facts of family medicine's situation. Most family doctors now work as employees. More are joining the employee ranks each day—narrowing their scope of work, reducing their autonomy, adopting a nine-to-five mentality, and avoiding long-term relationships with patients. It moves them further away from the generalist physician definition and toward a different definition: that of a primary care doctor who does only a smaller component of the kind of comprehensive care the generalist ideal embodies. Overall, the health system in the United States is still not tilting its axes in favor of either primary care or family doctors—regardless of the continued rhetoric spewed in one form or another, that is, getting health care costs under control, keeping people healthier, improving quality, and getting people better access to care. Other types of doctors have not embraced the patient management role of the family doctor, nor do they overtly advocate for it with their patients. The perception remains that many family doctors are jacks-of-all-trades, masters of none.

What is worse, family doctors as a collective are more balkanized and less cohesive than ever. We've seen that in the previous chapters. There is a sense among those in the field that something is not right about the specialty. Some feel there is a bait-and-switch aspect to becoming a family doctor. It ends up being something much different than what they were initially told. Others feel it is an impossible job to do well. The ask is too big for them. Still others believe sincerely in the ideal definition of the role, that of the generalist or comprehensive doctor, but find themselves working too hard or sacrificing too much to get it done. They find other niche-oriented ways to convince themselves they are doing "true" family medicine work. Family doctors everywhere are searching out more sustainable career paths for themselves, leading to so much career variety that the very label *family doctor* starts losing its preferred connotation.

What does the public think? This book has so far only addressed that constituency indirectly. But it merits some attention in this last chapter. After all, it is the public that has had more to do with family medicine remaining stagnant as a medical field than any other stakeholder—let's be honest. As Dr. Gayle Stephens astutely noted, people have been generally confused by the notion of a family doctor, one who is also a "specialist." There is no *Marcus Welby, M.D.* on television anymore to help show people, even in an ideal sense, what a family doctor can do. There are few doctors like Dr. Richard Rutland walking the earth today. More primary care is now done in big-box stores, urgent care centers, pharmacies, and big corporate health systems (Jonas 2018). Amazon and Apple may deliver primary care to us. More primary care in the future will be done through smartphones, tablets, and apps. Through these access points, family doctors either are not used or are severely limited in what they can do. Insurance plans are structured to allow patients to switch their doctors at will, which does not inspire loyalty. Primary care physician offices remain the highest cost access points for primary care, mostly due to the high labor cost of family doctors. Many primary care physician offices, with family doctors at the helm, still make it impossible for patients to feel welcome, with their long wait times for appointments and insertion of other non-physician providers between family doctor and patient. They simply do not understand how they are contributing to their own death spiral by removing themselves further from patients and generally annoying them.

Chances are most people in many parts of the United States do not have good opportunities to either see firsthand what a comprehensive family doctor does or develop a longer-term relationship with one. Take me, for example. I have burned through several family doctors over the past decade despite wanting to establish a relationship with one. All worked as employees for larger organizations. All had very limited scopes of practice. The benefit of having any sort of long-term relationship with any of them never really materialized. Their offices closed at 5 p.m. They were impossible to get timely appointments with, and most of the time, I was pawned off on their nurse practitioners or other doctors that had open appointment slots. When an emergency arose, they were never conveniently able to help me address the situation. I ended up going to urgent care centers more because I discovered those places could also meet many of my primary care needs. Most of the family doctors with whom I have interacted as a patient seem like nice people. They're all pretty good doctors too I would imagine. But the mutual loyalty was not there. There was no sense of comprehensiveness when it came to my care. I never sensed they cared much about me as a patient or a person trying to stay healthy. Because they saw me infrequently at best, this is not surprising.

That is the way it is for most of us, I would imagine; it's certainly that way for most of my family and friends. As if this was not bad enough, family doctors are increasingly hard to find. Those that are established often take no new patients. Those starting out in a traditional, office-based practice are few and far between. Increasingly, most primary care practices are employing nurse practitioners and physician assistants to take on new patients. That's good for their short-term bottom line because these non-physician providers are cheaper to employ, but it is a big mistake otherwise. It continues to create distance between family doctors and patients. In addition, there are competitors. For example, there are a fair number of general internal medicine practices still around in many parts of the country, and many people choose to go to those doctors, believing they know more clinically than the family doctor. Yes, the external environment of reimbursement and support for family doctors is not good, but the specialty needs to stop using that as an excuse for why it is failing with the public and young medical students.

Even with the number of challenges the specialty faces, all is not lost yet. But changes will need to be made. What family medicine looks like in twenty years will have to be meaningfully different from what it has tried to look like for the past fifty years. If primary care in the United States is to remain viable, with doctors delivering care and helping communities get healthier at its core, then it needs a larger army of generalist physicians to flood the country and practice the kind of medicine Nicholas Pisacano and Gayle Stephens envisioned. But it must be an adaptable army, not one that requires its members to adopt the unflinching definition of the all-encompassing patient management specialist. That brand has not sold well. That doctor will be hard to recreate in large numbers moving forward. It is perhaps neither practical from a system perspective or easy from a training perspective.

Family doctors must also be prepared to share their patients with technology, because technology will be able to manage a number of patient needs in the future better than any single family doctor. The COVID-19 pandemic has brought telemedicine to the fore. More primary care will be done virtually in the future. That fact is not the end of the world for family doctors; it is merely the reality they will need to accept moving forward. They will need to be ready to connect with their patients more frequently in real time. They will need to utilize instantly accessible smartphone apps that can integrate patient information in one place and help patients make decisions by filtering that information through machine learning algorithms. They will need to accept the aid of big tech companies like Apple and Amazon that know how to act as middlemen in a marketplace and that bring buyers and sellers together in ways they control. They will need to adopt integrated tech platforms that share patient information widely and strive to make patient management a fully collaborative venture. This is the future of patient management, and family doctors can work to put themselves at the center of this techno-logical revolution.

But if family doctors insist on trying to retain full control over the patient management aspect of the primary care equation, then that role will eventually be automated out of existence for them. If they turn their back on telemedicine because the reimbursement for it is not enough, they will lose out. Primary care as a part of the US health system is threatening to move away from an overreliance on physicians for many of its most mundane, standardized patient care activities. It will employ technology to market different services to patients and deliver some forms of primary care, use big data extensively to segment patients into disease-similar groupings and determine population or community health strategies, and prefer cheaper forms of labor who may also es-tablish relationships with patients. It will deliver on-demand primary care to people's homes, likely at a much more affordable price than now. All these things will potentially lessen the influence and power of the individual family doctor who provides a higher-cost version of primary care medicine. But how much so depends on if family doctors can do something to counter these trends.

There are no magic bullets to save family practice. But what if there were? What if we could identify several strategic steps that could be taken which, collectively, might transform the field and family doctors into something better aligned with the realities of the health care sys-tem now and in the future? What if we could give the specialty a leg up on competing against big tech and the Amazon effect in primary care? What if we could reinvigorate this physician army to better serve on the front lines of the war to make primary care victorious in America? The strategic steps that need to be taken may include some things that at first seem traumatic to do, but which offer long-term fixes for key problems noted in this book; other things that would be less traumatic but require meaningful changes in how family doctors are trained or how they work; and still other things that might not appear to be very big or important, but which, if committed to over time and with sustained tactical actions, could strike at the very heart of the question, how useful is a family doctor for patients?

A Top-Ten List for Saving Family Doctors

As a huge David Letterman fan back in the day, I always loved the top-ten lists on his show each night. Often read by a guest celebrity, these lists poked fun at many different aspects of life and were the perfect end to a stressful workday. That way of looking at the world (that everything can be boiled down to a list) has become part of our cultural lexicon. Another part of the lexicon is attaching probabilities to things that could happen in the future. Sportswriters in particular love doing this, writing article after article that speculate on the probabilities for where different free agents might sign, which teams will make the playoffs, and how college draft decisions will get made.

In the spirit of these two approaches to simplifying complex realities, here is a top-ten list, and their expected probabilities, for saving family medicine. They are not scientifically compiled but rather determined by me and based on what is in this book, my own knowledge of health care and primary care, and plenty of conversations I have had with family doctors over the years, as well as some research findings and survey results sprinkled in here and there. Take them for what they are worth. I would argue they are worth as much as anyone else's musings about how to make things better for the specialty and its doctors. There have been many efforts undertaken over the past several decades which have derived their own lists, efforts that were given lots of resources and brain power to come up with a plan.

How has that worked out so far?

Number Ten: Family Doctors Should Fully Embrace Virtual Care with Their Patients
Probability of Happening: Definitely More Likely

This one is a no-brainer. If family doctors were not beginning to seriously consider the use of things like telemedicine in their practice before, the COVID-19 pandemic pushed many of them to do it sooner rather than later. They had no choice. When the pandemic hit the United States in March 2020, many primary care offices across the country shut down for several months, seeing very few if any patients in person. Many offices continued to see only a limited number of patients in-office even after they had reopened (Larry Green Center 2020). In response, more family doctors have turned to telemedicine, both as a tactic to stay financially solvent and to get selected patients needed care (Shachar et al. 2020).

A recent survey of eight hundred doctors done before the pandemic, most of whom were primary care physicians, showed that telehealth use has begun to increase meaningfully over the past several years (Amwell 2019). For example, 15 percent of physicians in this survey said they used telehealth several times or more per week for patient visits, and almost half of respondents said they used it at least a couple times or more a month. Only 3 percent of them said they would not use it into the future. Another survey of over fifteen hundred family doctors, conducted in 2015, showed that 90 percent of them would use telemedicine if they were compensated adequately for it (Business Wire 2015).

Poor reimbursement for telemedicine visits has always been the main stumbling block to family doctors using it more. The pandemic changed all that, at least temporarily. Payers such as Medicare, Medicaid, and private insurers provided reimbursement "parity" during the early months of the pandemic, allowing family doctors to receive similar compensation for telemedicine visits as they would for in-person patient visits (Centers for Medicare and Medicaid Services 2020; Schoenberg 2020). Family doctors, seeing revenue from in-person visits plummet, have turned quickly to using telemedicine to deliver chunks of their care. I recently interviewed some family doctors who are using telemedicine, and I was amazed to find how pleasantly surprised many of them are with the value of using it for patient care. Some saw benefits in building stronger relationships with their patients. Some said they could provide forms of care in areas like mental health in ways they could not do when visits were purely face-to-face. Some thought it was efficient for a lot of normal patient complaints. Whether this is a permanent trend or just a temporary blip remains to be seen. If payers reduce the compensation for telemedicine, undoubtedly many family doctors would likely abandon its use.

But that would be a mistake on their part. They should view it as a loss leader for enhancing their value with patients. They see that it has value for connecting with their patients, increasing both convenience and access to their offices—two things that we know modern family doctors have struggled with providing (Amwell 2019). It would help family doctors stay involved in their patients' pursuit of health and wellness. They could be more available to answer their patients' questions, talk to them about a health issue, or help them make a health care decision. Familiarity breeds trust, and by virtually connecting more with patients, family doctors would have more opportunities to develop and maintain trust with their patients.

This additional availability could also give family doctors greater legitimacy and control with patients. Call it patient management if you want, but I don't view this as family doctors doing the unpleasant work they don't like to do, the paperwork of specialty referrals and insurance authorizations; I view it as family doctors once again becoming the trusted advisors to their patients—keeping in touch with them on a regular basis through virtual means and being available for them when they need it.

Trust is a critical word to understand here. One of the ways a greater embrace of technology by family doctors could help preserve their futures in the health care system is by offering opportunities for trust-building with large numbers of patients who need to have greater faith in the health care system. That can be achieved by increasing the number of contact points over time—allowing more patients to know their doctor, and their doctor to know them. Gallup has tracked the US public's confidence in the health care system for several decades. What it consistently finds is that most of the public thinks the system is in a state of major crisis, that there are significant problems that must be solved. While it is often said that most people think kindlier of their own doctors than the system, the fact is that many of us increasingly feel overwhelmed by a health care system that is too fragmented, impersonal, and expensive (Hoff 2017).

Enter family doctors. By embracing technologies that put them in closer contact with their patients, they can reassert their claim to being the best advocate for patients. Trust is built through the strengthening of relational bonds between people. Telemedicine can help with this so long as it is not the only means by which doctor and patient interact over time—too much proven good comes from a strong human-to-human, face-to-face connection in health care. Trust between provider and patient leads to greater empathy, mutual respect, listening, honesty, and compliance (Hoff 2017). Using communication technologies that put family doctors in closer, more frequent contact with patients is certainly not the only thing that can build trust. But it can be a key ingredient.

Telemedicine is only one piece of the technology puzzle for family doctors. Much more is coming on the horizon that family doctors could use to their advantage. For example, Apple's new integrated health record, now in use in the Veterans Health Administration, is a harbinger of things to come—smartphone apps that allow patients to see their complete health care records in one convenient location (Williams 2020). But access to more of our health care information will not necessarily make us healthier without someone trained to help us integrate, interpret, and make decisions with it. Family doctors can serve in that role. Of all physicians, they are still in the best position to act as our health care information consultants. They want to get paid what they think they are worth to do it, though, and I do not blame them. The problem with the kind of primary care tech companies push is that it likely will not pay family doctors in accordance with what they think they deserve to get paid. But if they pass on this opportunity, simply because they are not getting the compensation they want, you can be sure some machine learning chat bot or corporate behemoth like CVS Health, Apple, or Amazon will be there waiting to assume that role. For far less money too.

How likely is it that family doctors and the specialty of family medicine will embrace communications technology and virtual care delivery to connect significantly with their patients on a permanent basis? I give it a 75 percent chance, which among all the things on this top-ten list makes it the most likely to happen. Why such a high chance? Well, the optimism must be somewhere. This is low-hanging fruit that does not require a lot of pain on doctors' part, especially now that the pandemic has sped up what might have taken several more years to happen. Maybe I am wrong. There is no doubt many doctors do not want patients having real-time access to them, and they definitely want to get paid appropriately for that access.

Will patients want to do it? I think so, especially after this pandemic is over. I had my first telehealth visit recently and thought it was great. At the very least, they will see it as a valuable compliment to in-person care delivery. It may end up being more affordable too. Of course, some will be better able than others to play their part in this endeavor. All things being equal, most of us generally prefer to interact with doctors if it is convenient and not too expensive to do so. We also need our own technological tools and savvy to be able to do it virtually. But if family doctors cannot embrace this idea, many of the other strategic steps on this top-ten list stand an even lower chance of coming to fruition.

Number Nine: Remain the Patient's Chief Data Sentinel
Probability of Happening: Could Happen but Less Likely

This one is a tall order, which is why I give it a smaller chance of happening. While family doctors may not have control over this becoming a reality, there is no doubt that one key to greater power and relevance for family doctors is the ability to oversee the use and distribution of patient information, particularly when those doctors have established relationships with their patients. Why do you think companies like Amazon, Google, and Apple are spending so much time now trying to acquire patient information and become its purveyors (Landro 2020)? It's because patient information is big business. Having authority over patient health information and being at the center of the flow of clinical information between different stakeholders in the health care system—patients, insurers, other specialists, and community-based organizations that deal in health care or social service delivery—makes it possible to monetize that information by offering new products and services to patients and others who deliver care. It forces others to go through you to get that information.

Admittedly, given how much disruption is occurring in primary care, it is difficult to imagine family doctors functioning as the central information brokers for the primary care delivery system. First, there is already an electronic health record for almost all patients in America that makes the potential for information to be shared and accessed widely. This patient information will soon be stored fully in the cloud-based products of different technology companies, where it can be accessed and shared much more easily. Second, there is an accepted belief now that, at least in theory, patients should own their health information and have the right to make decisions about who should have access to it and how. Third, there is a belief that others simply can do it better than physicians from a technological standpoint. Large tech companies like Apple, Google, and Amazon seek to establish their own dominance as the hubs of health information, using their cloud services and their smart devices like Alexa and the iPhone (Williams 2020). All these companies do is deal in customer data. It is at the core of their business model. The thinking goes that they can position themselves and their gadgets closer to patients than doctors can, that is, right in the middle of their living rooms. For these companies, controlling patient health information is key to their strategic goals of becoming "market makers" in health care—bringing service providers and patients together, creating services and products to sell directly to patients, and trying to become trusted sources of advice for patients (Williams 2020).

By and large, patients do not trust large corporations to protect their information (Politico and Harvard T.H. Chan School of Public Health 2019). They may not trust physicians or their offices that much either. But at least in one recent survey, they trust their doctors more than hospitals or insurers (Politico and Harvard T.H. Chan School of Public Health 2019). This is where family doctors can try and gain an upper hand. This is the weak spot in the tech company armor. Traditionally, physicians were the chief stewards over our medical records. Before the electronic health record, our information sat in the doctor's office, recorded on paper in folders that sat on shelves behind the receptionist's desk. Though the paper record was fraught with problems ranging from incomplete information to missing information to illegible information, it was relatively secure in only one place, the doctor's office. Yes, we could not get at it easily as patients. But no one else could either. Of course, another problem with the paper record method was the inability of patient information to travel quickly across the health care system. This lent to greater service fragmentation, more chance for medical errors, and additional inconveniences for patients who needed to see or transfer their information to other doctors.

To save their specialty, family doctors must once again assert their legitimate right to act as the chief sentinels, along with patients, over this information. Here is the pitch: "Would you want Amazon or Facebook to know that you have a sexually transmitted disease or Alzheimer's disease, or would you rather that information stay private between you and your doctor?" With the major patient privacy law, the Health Insurance Portability and Accountability Act (HIPAA), now amenable to having technological devices like Amazon's Alexa become HIPAA compliant, meaning that they can serve as communication platforms for patient information (Krasniansky 2019), the floodgates will open for other non-physician organizations to receive the same approval soon enough. With patient records moving into the cloud at a faster pace, it will not be long before family doctors become just another customer vying for the right to access them.

One can clearly envision a future, if these changes are left unchecked, where Alexa or some other device interacts with us in our home, answering our health-related questions, diagnosing our symptoms, offering treatment advice, and recommending next steps in where to go for additional care. Make no mistake, in this future family doctors are largely cut out of the initial patient evaluation. They may see a patient downstream once Alexa tells that patient to visit a doctor's office, but they will now have Alexa and Amazon between themselves and the patient, further weakening the patient's loyalty to them. They will be cut out of the initial important decisions patients have to make about when and where to access health care. Machine learning algorithms will help patients make those first decisions. Patients will come to rely on this technology to help them figure out what to do, filter and make sense of their health information, and get it from one place to the other. Don't believe that? Just think how much you rely on your smartphone and its apps now to tell you what to do or how to do it. When was the last time you used a paper map to get somewhere?

What kinds of patient data should family doctors and their professional associations fight harder to control? Most importantly, the clinical data that describes a patient's health status: lab and imaging test results, diagnostic data of all types, physical exam findings, and treatment regimens. Second, personal information that is pertinent to a patient's health status, such as family histories, demographic characteristics, lifestyle information, and living situations—the sensitive personal information that all of us do not want public. Technology companies want this information so they can monetize it by creating services and products to sell to customers. Family doctors should want it so that they can serve as the patient's trusted partner in protecting this information, helping to decide who gets to see it, and how it is used for the patient's health care decision making.

It would take legislation and regulation to enable family doctors to serve in this role, and to minimize the potential role of other players like the tech giants. It would take a concerted lobbying effort by the specialty, and one hell of a marketing campaign, to even have a chance. Finally, it would take individual family doctors seeing the wisdom of fighting to get more authority as the patient's partner in protecting their health care data. What is this wisdom? In part, it involves family doctors adopting a loss-leader-type attitude (again, see the last recommendation) that acknowledges that they will gain additional power and relevance in the health care system if not extra time or pay. They will also gain the patient's trust.

The medical profession, and individual doctors, usually do not like to do anything for free. Given the heavy workloads many family doctors are under, and their status as employees of larger health care organizations, they may have neither the motivation nor agency to act in this role. Granted then, it is a long shot. But whoever it is that becomes the patient's partner with respect to helping them manage and use their health care information, that person or organization or company immediately takes one step closer to gaining the patient's loyalty and dependence on their service. In that respect, it should be on the list of things to help save family medicine.

Number Eight: Make Patients Your Partners
Probability of Happening: Could Happen but Less Likely

This one should have more than a 50 percent chance of happening, and that's because it is another no-brainer. But the lower expectation of it happening across the entire specialty of family practice is based mainly on the animal with whom we are dealing with here, namely, doctors. Doctors gravitate toward words like *power*, *control*, and *authority*. Lawyers, professors, engineers, and airline pilots do too—really, all elite professionals trained to believe they are the chosen ones like these words. They are less fond of words such as *partner* or *collaborator*. This comes from their training and socialization, the changing of which (spoiler alert!) is listed further down in this top-ten list.

What does "making the patient your partner" mean? Above all else, it means including the patient as an important part of the primary care health team, which also includes the family doctor, their assistants, and perhaps others (e.g., social workers and visiting nurses) from whom the patient receives services. The word *team* is used with reckless abandon in health care, so much so that it comes to mean nothing specific in most instances. What I mean here is that the patient should be treated as much as possible as a *co-equal* and full collaborator when it comes to making decisions in the primary care space. Patients should be given all relevant information about their situations. They should be talked to by family doctors and others on the health care team as if they are ultimately in control of all decisions. Their opinions and knowledge should be listened to and respected. They should advocate, together with the rest of the health care system, for the things that matter, such as the right to control their own medical information. This idea is not new. It has been advocated for in health care for decades.

Of course, the pushback to this idea is the notion that "patients really do not want to be involved in their care." This is a classic physician line meant to rebut the harder realization that comes from appreciating what must be done to be true partners with your patients. Some of what must be done is mentioned above: establish and maintain a good ongoing relationship; build trust; be available often and in real time; embrace different ways of communicating; be a steward of the patient's information and help guard its access by others; consider the patient's perspective and treat it with respect; be ready to modify your own expert decision making with the needs, wants, and preferences of the patient; fight for your patients' rights in the community and in their workplace. These things help to improve the chances patients will get more involved in their care, as a recent review of the literature showed (Vahdat et al. 2014). They also help improve outcomes (Hoff 2017).

This is hard work. No one is denying that. It is made harder by an inhospitable health care delivery setting with low reimbursements for activities like listening, a primary care system bent on copying Amazon to speed up service delivery, and insurance plans that require patients to make careful decisions about how and where to spend their out-of-pocket dollars. They are also made harder by the push to make family doctors efficient and by the presence of family doctors who embrace values that see medicine like a job rather than a calling. This book has already analyzed this litany of issues that stand in the way of this top-ten list of recommendations being adopted.

The patient as partner is good medicine. The research shows this well. The hope is that good medicine will be seen by patients as something in which their family doctor is involved. Once recognized for it, the value of the family doctor is elevated for those patients. This is not wishful thinking. A study of primary care doctors I did for a book several years ago showed this firsthand (see Hoff 2017). I interviewed several dozen patients about their experiences with primary care doctors, many of whom were family doctors. What I found was that where the doctor-patient relationship, through the eyes and experiences of the patient, was strong, and had many of the features noted above, the perceived value of that doctor was greater. The loyalty to those doctors by patients was greater. The desire to comply with mutually agreed upon clinical decisions was greater.

Where a strong doctor-patient relationship was not present, and where the patient did not feel in partnership with the doctor, the perceived value, loyalty, and compliance were all lower. Patients felt, when they were not treated as partners, that the difference between going to a primary care doctor's office and going to a retail clinic or urgent care center was negligible. For many of them, going to a primary care physician's office was a bigger hassle and not worth the extra time, effort, and potential money. When I spoke with primary care doctors in that same study, all agreed that they needed to have strong bonds with patients to make the relationship work. That relationship required mutual trust and respect. But many of them still cited outside forces as the main reasons such a partnership did not evolve. In other words, it was not their fault. The need for personal responsibility in making it happen was talked about less.

This is problematic because this one falls largely on the shoulders of individual family doctors. It requires a lot of personal effort, time, and willingness to put up with some major hassles that should not be minimized but should also not become blanket excuses. The fact is that many (not all) patients these days want to be heard. The retail tactics seeping into the health care industry, for better or worse, seek to "activate" the patient as a consumer, with the idea being that they become engaged in the services and products they receive from their doctors and the health care system (Hoff 2017). Family doctors may have problems seeing their patients as "consumers" (Hoff 2020), yet that is the way of the world now in most industries. For these reasons, I put the likelihood this recommendation comes to fruition at 40 percent. Unfortunately, it might take another generation before it can be realized, which might be too late for family medicine.

Number Seven: Organize Locally and Create Small Advocacy Armies for Family Doctors
Probability of Happening: More Likely than Not

Here is the thing—the way family doctors are organized collectively in 2020 is out of step with the interests they need to advocate for, which are job and workplace specific, and the realities of their employment arrangements. This is not news to many of us. I did a study and published an article about it twenty years ago, where I said doctors had to find new ways to push their interests in organizations (Hoff 2000). It continues to be news not heeded by the traditional powers in medicine. The outdated structure of having one's professional association at the federal, state, and local levels also serve as the default vehicle for family physician advocacy at the local level does not make sense anymore. Professional associations fight mainly over things like who can do the work and assuring the competency of those who do that work. They fight for professional autonomy. They are much less proficient in advocating for the kinds of things that employees need and want: good treatment from their employer, fair compensation and benefits, job satisfaction, reasonable workloads, and, some voice in how their jobs are structured.

Most family doctors are now, or will become, salaried employees. Many of today's barriers standing in the way of family doctors enhancing their value to patients and being comprehensive physicians stem from this reality. They can be hired and fired by their employers. Their work schedules and what they get paid are controlled by their employers. These employers also divvy up the work of family doctors into fragmented pieces. This raises issues about how these doctors are treated by their employers, their lack of workplace control, and how their jobs are structured. Just look at the recent COVID-19 pandemic and the realities many frontline physicians had to deal with, including a lack of personal protective equipment, little say in their working conditions, and being placed in unsafe situations (Ramos et al. 2020).

The traditional medical professional association seeks to keep the public, payers, and policy makers bought into the notion of the physician as an elite, independent expert, separate from any organization or corporation. To that end, these associations maintain the atmosphere of an exclusive club through the structuring of medical education and control over continuing medical education, advocating policies to protect the physician's power vis-à-vis other non-physician providers, and setting the rules for licensing requirements. No doubt, these are important arenas for maintaining professional control in health care.

But where professional associations remain largely ineffective is in locally representing different groups of doctors, each of which may be subject to unique job and employment circumstances. In addition, what is the point of being the primary clinical decision maker for patients when you have to comply constantly with edicts and guidelines that your employer or the patient's insurer make you follow? One reason why professional associations are ineffective is the fact that they do not wish to call out the reality that many doctors, family doctors especially, have lost significant power to the larger health care corporation. As we saw, most family doctors coming out of residency work as employees. They own nothing. They cede control on many fronts to their employers. Even older family doctors, like Orrin, who may have at one time owned their own practices, find themselves selling those practices or moving into highly dependent economic relationships with larger health systems, remaining "owners" in name only.

To acknowledge family doctors as another group of employees, albeit highly trained and compensated ones, would be a strategic mistake in the eyes of their professional associations. For an association like the American Academy of Family Physicians, advocating for family doctors in the same ways nurses and social workers are advocated for is a risky proposition. It might undermine the traditional message that family doctors are elites who are able to call their own shots. But family doctors no longer call their own shots in the workplace. They have not for some time. Many now have more in common with nurses and social workers.

The need for organizing locally among family doctors has never been stronger or more relevant to their future survival. Some of the stories from family doctors in this book highlight this point. Now, certain family doctors reading this might respond, "so do you mean organizing into a *union*?" The u-word has always been anathema to organized medicine in the United States. The most well-known physician union in the United States, the Union of American Physicians and Dentists, was formed way back in 1972, yet it is still centered primarily on the West Coast and remains small, with only several thousand members (Union of American Physicians and Dentists 2020).

The notion that professionals like doctors are not allowed to unionize or collectively bargain for wages or employment conditions has been supported legally for decades through various court decisions. In large part, the logic is that physicians are de facto "supervisors" of other workers in the health care setting, thus making them "management" rather than "employees." However, with most physicians now regarded as employees who have no managerial duties to speak of, and reduced control over clinical decision making, opportunities to collectively bargain within different organizations should become more legally challengeable. Even so, I am not even talking about needing to organize into a union here. What I am talking about is any organizing vehicle, formal or informal, that could encourage family doctors sharing similar work settings and jobs to come together with the intent of sharing their experiences, developing collective-action agendas, and supporting each other in the drive to make their everyday work lives more fulfilling and their value to patients greater.

Perhaps the word *guild* is better to use here. For centuries, guilds have been used as a combined professional association and trade union for craftspersons such as merchants, masons, blacksmiths, plumbers, and electricians. A guild simply refers to a form of collective organization that allows an occupational group to advocate for and protect its interests. Family doctors need to consider developing local organizations that are more in the spirit of the guild concept. They should be localized to the specific health care organization, job, or work setting. Even if unable to bargain collectively over formal employment contracts with their employers, such local groups could provide counterpressure to health care organizations—which in turn might make the latter include the family physician's voice more in their decision making.

These local family doctor guilds could be used for any and all of the following: (a) trying to make employers aware of deleterious workplace conditions; (b) pushing back on requirements that impede the family doctor's workday, such as in areas like quality improvement; (c) seeking greater collaboration in how work schedules and workloads for family doctors, and the entire health team within a setting, are organized; (d) advocating for specific patient care issues; and (e) seeking employment-related benefits such as fair and equal pay, transparent promotion and reward structures, benefits to promote appropriate work-life balance, and continuing education.

I put the probability this recommendation is adopted at about 60 percent. There is no doubt family doctors will grow amenable to the idea of local collective organizing, which makes me optimistic. Just listen to the many voices in this book. Physicians are trained in many ways to be independent, and many who self-select into medicine as a career are loner types. Their professional associations likely will not help in the endeavor, and the organizations for whom they work may seek to challenge legally some of what might be done in this regard. No matter. Soon enough, I predict the legal protections for physicians to organize, the way nurses do, will be granted. The long and short of it, and why this recommendation makes the list: if family doctors do not gain some greater localized form of collective representation, their working conditions will continue to worsen and their voices will become more muffled. That undercuts the specialty's survival prospects.

Number Six: Create Strategic Alliances with Other Health Occupations and Competitors
Probability of Happening: As Likely as Not

If you were to ask me if I thought this recommendation was realistic right now, I would say no. But over the next decade, as primary care in the United States, and elsewhere for that matter, succumbs to the lack of available physicians, it must come to pass. What do I mean by it? I mean that family doctors must seek out greater partnerships with both non-physician occupations and other medical specialties—strategic alliances to advance what, as noted under the previous recommendation, are increasingly common interests. Non-physician occupations include nurse practitioners and physician assistants. Other medical specialties include hospitalists—doctors who take care of patients only while they are in the hospital—and emergency medicine physicians—doctors who take care of patients only while they are in emergency rooms or urgent care centers. The very groups of doctors that cut into the family doctor's business decades ago.

For family doctors, these types of partnerships should be aimed at enhancing their control over the primary care delivery system. For example, achieving the role of chief data sentinel for patients' medical information is aided by enhanced communication and information exchange with delivery settings where their patients are found and where primary care is delivered. These other settings include urgent care centers, retail clinics, and hospitals where all these potential partners work, and where many family doctors do not work. Becoming the proverbial patient-knowledge hub in the wheel of primary care delivery might give family doctors and their offices enhanced ability to compete more effectively with the big-box stores, hospitals, and pharmacy chains that now seek to put themselves between these doctors and their patients. They may be less likely to be kept out of the patient care loop. But they must have the cooperation of the providers that work in these settings.

In terms of greater local collective advocacy, forging relationships with other groups of providers who also need such advocacy could increase the family doctor's ability to be heard against the din of the larger health care corporation that now wants to guide the narrative patients in US health care hear (Hoff 2017). That prevailing narrative minimizes the need for a primary care doctor at the center of a patient's care. Imagine nurse practitioners and physician assistants, allied with family doctors, and even patients, pursuing better working conditions for themselves, greater autonomy, and improved patient care. Imagine how much more relevant different groups of primary care "providers" become if they speak as one collective voice and advocate in such a way as to give their employers little room to play one group against the other.

It will take some doing to get family doctors to treat these other occupations as co-equals and to allow them some degree of practice freedom in return for helping them strengthen their roles as comprehensive physicians. Right now, the American Academy of Family Physicians (AAFP), the voice of family doctors in America, would prefer to keep those occupations under their thumb. That is not a smart move. From the AAFP website:

> The AAFP position is that the term "nurse practitioner" should be reserved for those who undergo specific training programs following attainment of a Registered Nurse (R.N.) license. Following licensure as an R.N., the nurse desiring to function as a nurse practitioner should be certified rather than licensed as a nurse practitioner.
>
> The nurse practitioner should not function as an independent health practitioner. The AAFP position is that the nurse practitioner should only function in an integrated practice arrangement under the direction and responsible supervision of a practicing, licensed physician. In no instance may duties be delegated to a nurse practitioner for which the supervising physician does not have the appropriate training, experience and demonstrated competence. (American Academy of Family Physicians 2020b)

This is the problem with such a stance: saying nurse practitioners (NPs) should only be "certified" rather than "licensed" conveys a desire to keep them from doing patient care independent of family doctors, which the next paragraph goes on to say. But NPs already have independent practice ability in about half of US states, so that ship is sailing fast, whether family medicine likes it or not (American Association of Nurse Practitioners 2020). Big-box stores and chains like CVS Health see this cheaper and more controllable non-physician provider at the core of their new business model for fast, convenient primary care. The big issue is orienting family medicine to understand where this is all heading for them—getting them to accept the trade-offs in viewing NPs and physician assistants as able to provide good patient care without physician supervision. In return, they can gain an ally in the fight against their true enemy: the health care corporation—be it a hospital, health care system, or retail intruder like Amazon.

Where other medical specialties like hospital and emergency medicine are concerned, strategic alliances are a must moving forward. The reality is that family doctors had earlier opportunities to possibly absorb, or at the very least establish strong strategic alliances with, these specialties during their formation several decades ago. For instance, the field of family medicine had a chance to potentially make the field of emergency medicine part of their specialty in the mid-1970s. Much of who was doing what was called *emergency medicine* during that time were family doctors. That said, this never came to pass, and the specialty of emergency medicine had its own certification exam and specialty board by the early 1980s. Ironically, the current AAFP position is advocating for family doctors to practice emergency medicine without certifying in that specialty.

> Family physicians are trained in the breadth of medical care, and as such are qualified to provide emergency care in a variety of settings. Many family physicians currently provide quality emergency department and trauma care throughout the nation, including military, rural, and remote settings.
>
> Specialty certification alone should not prevent family physicians from practicing in any emergency setting or trauma center at any level. Emergency department credentialing should be based on training, experience and current competence. Combined residency programs in family medicine and emergency medicine, or additional training, such as fellowships in emergency medicine or additional course work, may be of added benefit. (American Academy of Family Physicians 2020a)

Formal collaboration agreements, shared training, reciprocity arrangements, and collective advocacy are all means by which the field of family medicine can unite with these other specialties to assert their interests and unique status (American Board of Family Medicine 2020). In this case, the strategic goals for family medicine are multiple. First, gain greater ability to train for and practice medicine in these other areas, to provide a wider array of sustainable employment and career opportunities for family doctors. Second, for those family doctors wishing to engage in the comprehensive physician role, create opportunities for them to interact with doctors caring for their patients in other settings, allowing them to maintain the patient management role in an organic way, one the patient will recognize and buy into.

Alliances with specialties like emergency and hospital medicine would, like the case of nurse practitioners and physician assistants, allow family doctors to sit at the nexus of care delivery for their patients, have a better chance to become the patient's chief data sentinel, and gain a stronger advocacy position for working conditions and patient care with their employers. In short, it would facilitate several other recommendations on this list. The goal is not to wrest control from physicians in other specialties. It is to increase their own relevance as generalist doctors able to manage their patients' care needs. In addition, many of the same issues plaguing family medicine, including burnout, excessive workloads, too much paperwork, and overly standardized care, also plague doctors in these other specialties. The interests across the specialties are increasingly shared. I believe many family doctors working on the ground understand the potential of becoming greater allies with these other stakeholders. But the 50 percent probability that this happens represents the historical territoriality that all medical specialties exhibit, even when it is counter to their own interests. Whether this happens in the next decade comes down to a coin flip.

Number Five: Expand the Work of Family Medicine Creatively and Relationally
Probability of Happening: Definitely More Likely

What does this recommendation mean? I am not fully sure. But one thing I do know is that unless family doctors "re-expand" their scope of work in creative ways, their value to patients and the health care system will continue to shrink. Primarily being patient managers will not cut it, as noted earlier in this chapter, for two reasons. First, patients do not want or value paper pushers who fill out forms and checklists, and that is what patient management means to health care organizations that employ family doctors. Mundane patient management does not thrill many young family doctors, as we have seen. It simply is more cost-effective to have non-physicians and tech gadgets do it. Second, the more elaborate patient management role requires being a true comprehensive or generalist family doctor, a role which many of these individuals may not fulfill.

The creative re-expansion of family doctor work should focus, in every aspect, on leveraging the *relational aspects* of care delivery. In other words, the things family doctors, as *humans*, can do that tech gadgets or artificial intelligence cannot do. They are things that involve expert, tacit knowledge: of patients' lives, of how local communities function, of how the local health care system works, and of how all these things come together to shape a person's health status. They are things that involve taking appropriate action in areas such as patient advocacy, bridge building within health care systems, emotional support for patients, and policy development and implementation. They are things that leverage knowledge of the individual patient and their circumstances.

Note what I am getting at here. This pivot to building a scope of work that has relational excellence woven throughout does not mean that each family doctor must have a broad scope of clinical practice in their everyday work. They do not really have to be doing comprehensive care delivery. That is the old, and frankly, wrong perspective to take when trying to save a specialty that has never claimed procedural domains for itself, and for which the public and payers have not bought into. What type of creative scope then? Here is one: how about community-oriented family health? What does this mean? It means work that integrates knowledge about the individual patient and their family with knowledge about their living situation, community supports, and the local health care system—all with an eye toward not only advancing the individual patient's health but also the community health infrastructure, as well as taking on the larger societal problems like poverty and racism that undermine people's health. This is the sort of work some of our true believers discussed in previous chapters were trying to do.

Now, the field of family medicine might say, "yes, all of our doctors are trained to do that, and they do it!" But in reality, they do not. If the smaller sample of family doctors interviewed for this book is any indication, very few family doctors pursue the consistent integration of individualized patient care with community or family health as a major part of their workday. Very few engage in local community advocacy, primarily on behalf of their patients, or seek to improve functioning of the surrounding health care delivery system. Now this is not true for every family doctor. But making this an expanded and formalized focus for some in the field would arguably increase the specialty's relevance, certainly in the communities where they practice, which is part of where family medicine has languished. That is, it has received less recognition of its value among the wider population of people in a geographic area.

Family medicine training would have to change, which is why that recommendation is next on the list. Except for a few residency programs here and there around the United States, family doctors are not provided with deep training and experiential opportunities in areas like community advocacy, health policy, or health systems management. Significant (i.e., not just a few months) business and practice-management training should be part of the family doctor's training for this expanded scope. Training in public health, policy analysis, community organizing, legislative advocacy, psychology, and social work should be included as well. Where will all this go? How is there enough space in the current training model to accommodate it? Create an extra residency year for every family doctor if you must. Or, better yet, look at medical school training and acknowledge that a good chunk of it is increasingly outdated, unnecessary, and not well aligned with creating real family doctors. Advocate for changes there.

These new and creative scopes of work, emphasizing relational medicine, can also be integrated into different clinical areas and settings in which family doctors are already working—the hospital, emergency room, urgent care center. Why not? The big assumption here, and I am convinced it does hold, is that regardless of where they seek treatment, patients benefit from knowing their doctor. Now the pushback is that no one will pay for a hospital or emergency room doctor, for example, to stay in contact with patients they only see episodically. But an increasing number of family doctors work for larger health systems and group practices that should have an interest in developing relationships with patients who are not their own but still come to them for acute care services. For them it is an opportunity to grab new business. For their existing patients, it is an opportunity to provide a richer customer experience.

There is a dearth of good relational medicine in all areas of health care: primary care, urgent and emergency care, hospital care, end-of-life care, community health, post-acute care, rehabilitation care, maternal and child health, geriatrics, and the list goes on. Expanding family practice scopes of work into the arena of relational medicine will create a range of additional career, work, and employment opportunities for family doctors. And it may get more medical students to pick family practice as a specialty choice. Because, as we have heard, they want options. Expanding relational scopes of work does not mean anyone in family medicine needs to become the type of comprehensive physician Richard Rutland and Marcus Welby represented. Family doctors can still work in a niche clinical area, but they'll become specialists in the relational components needed for patients in that area. A true commitment to the relational may create less cynical family doctors who feel betrayed once they are in practice—like Serena and Joanna who were discussed in earlier chapters—because what they were told is not what they end up experiencing (Joseph and Japa 2019).

Number Four: Change How Family Doctors Are Trained
Probability of Happening: As Likely as Not

Where to begin? How about with John Millis and his committee's famous report for the American Medical Association from the 1960s:

> What is needed and what the medical schools and teaching hospitals must try to develop is a body of information and general principles concerning man as a whole and man in society that will provide an intellectual framework into which the lessons of practical experience can be fitted. This background will be partly biological, but partly it will be social and humanistic, for it will deal with man as a total, complex, integrated social being. (Millis 1966, p. 52)

I am not sure medical training has realized this vision yet. In part because family practice training remains marginalized in medical schools and academic teaching hospitals. But it is more than that. There are parts of this recommendation that apply to how we train all young medical students, not only those who become family doctors. Medical school is a daunting environment for a young would-be professional. It contains all the potential for burnout, dissatisfaction, and career regret (Dyrbye et al. 2006; Hoff 2018). For some students, it provides negative experiences that involve harassment, discrimination, and bias (Witte et al. 2006). Every student, regardless of their ultimate medical specialty choice could use a more empathetic, respectful, and enriching four years of training. This negative training environment does not help to sell the specialty of family practice. By a student's fourth year in medical school, family practice may look like a consolation prize—a suboptimal career choice not rewarding enough for the several grinding years of less-than-fun schooling they received.

Unless you change the medical school experience for all students, and make it a more positive one, family practice indirectly gets the short end of the proverbial stick because these students seek more for their sacrifices—a specialty that has higher prestige, compensation, autonomy, and better working hours. I have spoken with lots of US medical students over the years who begin medical school thinking favorably about primary care and becoming a family doctor (Hoff 2010). By year three or four, after they have been put through the sausage grinder of a textbook-based curriculum and tons of multiple-choice tests, and after they have worked with wave after wave of high-powered, highly paid specialists who oversee their training, they do not look upon primary care careers as anything special or desirable.

The medical school curriculum, as pedagogically structured, does not favor students choosing family practice in droves. The first two years of primarily hard science–based training, taught not by primary care doctors but by specialists working in the school's affiliated academic medical center, does little to educate a young student on the potential joys and importance of family medicine (see Hoff 2010). There is little extended coursework in holistic, relationally oriented medicine, the lynchpin of the traditional family medicine definition. Little attention is paid to softer clinical areas such as chronic disease management, social and behavioral health, pediatrics, or geriatrics—all key areas of the generalist physician's work domain. Almost no training is given on the business aspects of medicine, population health, or community health. Instead, all the attention focuses squarely on getting students prepared to pass Step 1 of the US medical licensing exam, which everyone takes between years two and three, and which forms the crux of evaluation for residency programs to pick their candidates. This test focuses on the basic scientific knowledge that was crammed into the student's head during those first two years, such as anatomy, physiology, microbiology, and biochemistry.

It would be wholly unrealistic, in these final pages, to suggest that general medical school training will change any time soon in favor of getting more students immersed and interested in family practice. There is too much tradition, too much competition rooted in those Step 1 exams, and too much ambivalence in the medical profession toward primary care and family practice to think that those first two years of training will be reformed quickly or significantly. What is left? For one, the clinical rotations students do in year three of medical school include a rotation in family practice. I have heard many young doctors and medical students over the years complain about how poorly these rotations are set up in their respective schools. This poor setup includes limiting the family practice rotation to in-hospital safety net clinics where there is little continuity of care, many noncompliant patients, and heavy workloads of episodic primary care—in other words, the aspects of family practice that are less enjoyable. It can also include the use of burned-out, dissatisfied family physician mentors who work for the hospital and who end up conveying a negative image of the overworked family doctor to students. In addition, rotations in family practice, which last only a couple of months, never allow students to practice much relational medicine with the same patients over time, and they do not show students the full picture of what comprehensive family medicine is or what its rewards can be.

Moving these rotations into other less adversarial primary care delivery settings is one way to change training for the better. Of course, the reason such training is embedded primarily in academic medical centers is because of the imitation approach family practice took in copying the training model of other medical specialties. Hospital-based work looks more serious to the outside world and to the other specialties from whom family medicine has always sought to gain acceptance. As discussed earlier, this imitation approach helped to create a fire wall between the specialty's newest recruits and the family doctors, working in communities across the United States, who were doing the kind of work Richard Rutland did—practicing a generalist brand of medicine with patient populations with whom they had ongoing relationships.

Besides shifting the focus and location of third-year family practice rotations, aligning the family medicine residency experience with the kinds of careers, jobs, and scopes of work many younger family doctors now choose, and training them better in relational medicine from the outset, would have a greater bang for the buck. Traditionally, the first year of a family practice residency places a heavy emphasis on inpatient hospital care and clinical work that very few family doctors, if any, end up doing once out in full-time practice. It involves rotating family medicine residents, for a couple of months at a time, through different hospital-based services such as surgery, intensive care, emergency medicine, and obstetrics. These hospital-based rotations often only expose family practice residents to working with patients in episodic ways, either when patients are in the hospital or when they are visiting the hospital for certain services, so residents are not exposed to the kind of longitudinal patient care that family doctors practice.

Why is there so much emphasis on inpatient services during year one? The specialty's early focus on imitating how other clinical specialties were trained is one reason. Another related reason is that most family practice residency programs are based in or closely affiliated with hospitals. Could the first year of family practice residency emphasize primarily outpatient and community-based medicine? Could it connect residents more closely with those primary care physicians working in their own practices, to help them get exposed earlier and quicker to longitudinal patient relationships, patient management, and comprehensive care from the community family doctor perspective? Could developing relational skills gain prominence in that first year, creating a foundation for young family doctors to then take those relational skills and apply them in years two and three to specific work such as ambulatory care, hospital medicine, community health, population health, geriatrics, emergency medicine, or urgent care?

Of course, some family medicine residency programs around the country already experiment with "clinic first" models of training in which residents are exposed to longitudinal care with the same patients. But such models are still the exception rather than the norm in family practice residency training; they need to exist everywhere. They also tend to be centered within the walls of primary care clinics in academic medical centers, which is still not the best or most representative place to learn how to be a generalist family doctor. It is a hard place to learn the generalist trade. Their mentors in these settings are overworked, often-dissatisfied primary care teaching faculty who work for the academic medical center or hospital as salaried employees with little autonomy. These medical centers are also still not interested in doing comprehensive primary care as the centerpiece of their mission; rather, doing it is a way for them to feed patients to other parts of the hospital doing higher-cost services.

Young family doctors will tell you that too much of residency is rooted in the hospital, that this training convinces many of them to simply stay and work full-time in the hospital or in an urgent care center. It is what they learn how to do best during residency. It is the work environment in which they feel most comfortable. Through their residency work, many do not see the real work of a generalist family doctor, and most do not get a fair opportunity to develop their own patient panels, follow them over time, develop strong relationships with them, and be their comprehensive doctor. They get mentored by overworked family doctors who are often not the best examples for them to follow if they want to embrace a generalist role. This continues into years two and three of a residency. But at least during those later two years—if family practice residency training got more specialized and allowed residents to narrow their scope of residency training halfway through toward a niche area like hospital medicine, outpatient medicine, or urgent care—there would already be a strong background in relational medicine that could then be applied to any of these niche areas. This would allow young family doctors to "sub-specialize," while still possessing the relational and management skills needed to set themselves apart from everyone else.

That family practice residents are used as cheap labor, helping hospitals and academic medical centers make ends meet and care for the uninsured, is no secret. This is where the leadership of family medicine needs to see that the interests of their young trainees are not the same as the interests of their residency employers. My bet is they already know that. The structure of family medicine residencies remains a part of the deal with the devil the specialty, and leaders like Nick Pisacano, chose to make decades ago. That deal will not get renegotiated easily. The devil always wants his due.

Number Three: Temporarily Downsize Family Practice—Create Scarcity and Better Fit with Generalist Training Opportunities
Probability of Happening: Could Happen but Less Likely

This is a heretical recommendation from the point of view of family practice. It also seems counterintuitive. After all, the field gauged its popularity and success for decades on how fast it was growing, how many medical students were choosing it, and how many new residency programs were opening. In other words, the specialty was playing the numbers game and focusing on quantity over quality. But the numbers have never been in family practice's favor. We saw that in the last chapter. A consistent 12–15 percent of US medical school graduates have chosen family practice annually for the past fifty years, well short of the 25 percent goal. There have been an increased number of family practice residency positions available each year, but only about half of those positions are filled with graduates of US medical schools, leaving them to sit empty or be filled by international medical graduates or osteopathic students. Yes, it is a large specialty in terms of overall numbers of doctors, but that was also true for the field of general practice at one time, and raw numbers did not help that field survive.

Why not strategically decrease the number of family practice residency positions available each year, at least for a short five-to-ten-year window? By how many? That is not my call, but residency positions get similarly squeezed in many of the procedural specialties, even ones where patient demand runs high. Fields in high demand like dermatology rarely open their resident spigots to allow large increases in their numbers, even when demand from medical students and patients for that specialty is higher. They do that on purpose. Many of the procedural specialties proceed according to the Scarcity Principle, which states that the price of something goes up when it is in high demand and the available supply is low (Chen 2019). Long waits to see doctors like dermatologists make us as patients believe these clinical fields are more important, both for our health and in terms of financial value (i.e., what we think they should be paid). It makes medical students think these fields are the toughest to get into and the ones everyone values the most.

If there are fewer family doctors being turned out in the short term, I doubt that will make the current primary care access problems in the United States worse. Why? Because, as we have seen, many graduating family practice residents do not go into the kinds of jobs and work settings that would help ease the primary care shortage, nor do they go practice in the geographic locations (e.g., rural areas) where the shortages are most acute. They go to work in hospitals as hospitalists, in urgent care centers and emergency rooms as urgent care doctors. They take positions where they are not doing full-time outpatient medicine in a single practice setting. Many take outpatient medicine jobs in suburban and urban areas where the shortages are not as acute.

But there is another reason to promote temporary scarcity in the family practice specialty. It might allow the specialty to rightsize itself quicker toward creating more and better trained generalist family doctors. It could give more family practice residency programs a chance to move their training in a direction to create family doctors who do more things in their role. It might downsize or eliminate some of the more marginal family medicine residency programs that are short on available teachers and generalist teaching experiences. It might also allow for a sharper concentration of teaching and funding resources to fewer programs that have the best mentors who are committed to developing generalists, rather than developing family doctors who become hospitalists, urgent care doctors, or emergency room doctors.

Granted, this is a hard-core, self-interested strategic move. Yet the true numbers do not lie. Family practice struggles each year to get even half (in 2020 it was a third) of its annual first-year resident slots filled by US medical school graduates. That has been the norm for decades. There is no reason to think it will change without something that can trigger students and patients to think differently about its value. Of course, without following the previous recommendations, this one will probably not achieve what the Scarcity Principle dictates. But it is worth a shot. Would it accelerate the trend toward technology-based, non-physician-centric primary care talked about in an earlier chapter? Perhaps, but that is a risk worth taking for the specialty. There needs to be some overdue quality control in the family doctor production process, and to that end, there are probably more than a few family practice residency programs out there that should be closed or repurposed because they do not have the resources, faculty depth, or work settings to train residents in a high-quality manner. Squeeze the numbers for a few years and some of those programs will go away, which is probably not a bad thing.

Number Two: Rename and Rebrand the Family Medicine Specialty
Probability of Happening: Not Very Likely

Here goes—the most radical, at least from the perspective of the field, its true believers, and the many older family doctors who still believe primary care and family practice will make a comeback without having to do anything major: *rename and rebrand the specialty*. There, I said it. What is in a name? Everything, especially if it is one that has developed a negative or ambivalent connotation among key constituencies. If you doubt this, then you have not been reading this book, particularly the parts about the brand of general practice and how quickly that brand deteriorated. And how quickly the founders of family practice wanted to get away from the *general practice* name. That name went from one of prestige and positive connotations in one decade to something odious and dying in the next.

Family practice is not in that place brandwise. At least not yet. But it seems to be clear that the identity issue outlined in this story is affected by a name that does not convey anything specific or clear to medical students or the public. The data in this book make that point clear. At the outset, there were those who questioned calling it *family practice*. Gayle Stephens, as we heard at the end of the last chapter, thought the public got confused with the name changing from general practice to family practice. So did others. The adjective *family* was chosen for reasons I still cannot fully figure out, even after examining all the documents I did for this book. Yes, there were those who pushed for that label. There was affinity for a physician who could be like the old country doc and take care of everyone. There were those who believed that there was a science behind the notion of "family health." But why it had to be that name is still unclear. All I can conclude is that the term *family practice* had a nice ring to it. It seemed wholesome and nostalgic. It conveyed not only a focus on the individual patient but on their larger social networks as well, and perhaps people felt this helped convey the idea of comprehensive medicine. Or perhaps people thought that it would give these doctors the ability to stake out a claim over larger groups of patients by capturing the family node. Maybe it was just that no one could think of a better name, and no one wanted to keep calling it general practice.

The name *family practice* arguably does not work anymore. Many family doctors do not understand what it means. Young ones seem to feel undermined by it because they get attached to a label they think means one thing, only to find out it means something else. We saw that with young doctors like Joanna and Serena. How many early-career family doctors take care of entire families these days? Less than you think, especially when many are working in the kinds of settings and jobs already described. For the public, the identity of a family doctor remains problematic and elusive. As a patient, I also do not think that term aligns well with what it is I believe that kind of doctor should be doing for me. My family doctor does not take care of my entire family. She takes care of me.

What could a new name for this specialty be? I do not know for sure. Here is one thought though: what about renaming it *general practice*? That would be ironic, but it is the type of clinical practice these doctors are supposedly trained to perform. They have still been called *generalists* time and again over the years. Yes, the name had a bad connotation by the 1960s, but that was sixty years ago. How about calling it something like *everyday medicine*? Laugh if you want, but is that not the goal of such a doctor—to ideally manage a patient's total care and be aware of the patient's full range of needs? What about *relational medicine*? *Holistic medicine*? Could such labels not convey that the primary goal of this type of doctor is to be the one person in the health care system that makes a lasting human connection with the patient? How about *personalized medicine*—a name that conjures up a branch of doctoring where patients are treated as unique individuals? Perhaps a combination of these names might make sense.

Name changes can do wonders for a brand. Many companies have changed their names, either to get away from a poor reputation or to pitch themselves in a more attractive, innovative way, with a lot of success. Nike used to be Blue Ribbon Sports. Google was founded as a company called Backrub. Pepsi started out as Brad's Drink. Kentucky Fried Chicken simplified to KFC. Relentless was renamed Amazon. Sound of Music became Best Buy (Conradt 2017). Physicians have done this too. For example, hospitalists used to be called *inpatient physicians*. Name changes can stimulate a positive reappraisal of what it is an organization has to offer its customers. It can make customers forget the past. Sure, any name change can backfire, but there are many instances of successful rebirth with only a simple moniker adjustment.

I give this recommendation around a 10 percent probability of happening, at least over the short term. My sense from speaking with leaders in family practice and reading plenty about how the specialty has remained beholden to the labels of *family physician* and *family practice* is that it would be considered heresy to make a change. But I rest my case for a name change on the analysis in this book, particularly the problems of identity and brand recognition, what many family medicine leaders writing about the issues in the field have said themselves about the name over the years, and the fact that the existing name has done little to help grow the field's scope of work or the number of medical students choosing it each year.

Number One: Something Else Radical the Family Practice Specialty Can Think Up
Probability of Happening: Could Happen but Less Likely

I will state it plainly. In the end, there are certainly smarter minds that can and should work on doing something significant to reinvigorate family practice and assure its future survival. But will they, or will they continue to double down on the existing name and identity? Will they continue to form special committees and engage in years-long superficial examinations of what they could do to enhance their existing brand, or will they blow that brand up and start innovating outside-the-box? I am not confident that the specialty can engage in a deeper, more profound self-examination. When a specialty keeps defining itself pretty much the same exact way for fifty years, in the face of underwhelming success and real threats to its survival, it is hard to imagine something big will happen by their own hand. But it must happen, so I am giving the probability that it does a 25 percent chance on the hope that some group of family practice leaders, perhaps others like Nick Pisacano, will realize the gravity of the situation and move boldly to address it.

There it is—my top-ten list for saving family practice. I admit, it does not have a lot of tactical detail. The field's leaders should develop tactics, but the big-picture strategies need to come first. You may ask why the list does not deal with the reimbursement issue for primary care services. There have been several reimbursement ideas proposed for primary care, and they have all failed. Greater economic value for what family doctors do does not come before or without a number of these recommendations being pursued; it comes as a result of implementing them successfully.

As much as I have studied this field, I have not seen many of these recommendations put forth. Most of these would have to be done simultaneously to produce a significant effect. Some will say several of them have been discussed or tried in some form by the specialty. Sure, some may have been discussed by some group or leadership team somewhere, but none have been followed religiously and taken to their full extreme. Many of the recommendations on this list have not been tried to any meaningful extent. At best, half measures, incremental experimentation, and continued maintenance of the status quo have been tried in the background—small pockets of change that were never scaled up and which usually flamed out. That is the history of family medicine. Do all the recommendations make sense? Maybe not. Some do, though. For others, perhaps they are meant as the start of a critical dialogue about what else can and should be done. Thinking bigger and bolder is necessary for saving the specialty. Saving it is defined as making it a valuable, central, and popular brand of medicine for years to come. It does not have to grow at an unrealistic pace, but it has to grow. Whatever growth there is for defining success should be authentic and sustainable. More young medical students should want to become family doctors. More than the number now should want to practice generalist medicine. A large number of family doctors should be engaged in the kinds of activities and practice described in the recommendations and be enthusiastic about doing these things. The general public should have a clear sense of who family doctors are and what they can do. The family practice brand should be clearly understood. These are some of the criteria for success. All is not lost yet. But time is of the essence.

Coda: A COVID-Damaged Health Care System, Primary Care, and the Family Doctor

When I began researching and writing this book, the COVID-19 pandemic was a tragic event still many months from entering our lives. As the pandemic hit the United States in March 2020, and primary care offices across America shut their doors, it became apparent that business as usual for family doctors was in danger of being majorly disrupted. As I write this last chapter in October 2020, I grow more convinced that we are at a major tipping point in transforming primary care service delivery in the United States. The pandemic has significant implications for family practice. There will likely be a permanent new normal established post-pandemic for some primary care service delivery.

Can we speculate a bit more on this new normal? First, it is important to appreciate that some changes in the US primary care system (and arguably in primary care systems across the globe) occurring because of the pandemic have been on the verge of happening for years. These changes may either present opportunities for family doctors or further erode their relevance and value to patients. Take telehealth for example. For years, primary care physicians resisted engaging in telehealth care delivery with their patients. For example, a 2018 Deloitte survey of doctors showed less than 20 percent possessing the infrastructure and capabilities to conduct telehealth visits with their patients (Abrams et al. 2018). These doctors cited obstacles such as lack of appropriate reimbursement and licensing issues for not wanting to perform virtual care with their patients. In primary care at least, very little virtual care was performed pre-pandemic.

That has changed for many family doctors, as noted above in one of my recommendations for saving family medicine. Telehealth became a means in 2020 for continuing to provide care to patients and earn needed revenues for family doctors and their employers (Schoenberg 2020). Its usage in primary care shot up for several months, then leveled off again as many doctors went back to the traditional model of in-person visits. This return to the old way of doing things is not advisable for family doctors. Telemedicine in primary care is here to stay. The pandemic sped up the implementation of that innovation more in a few months than in the entire decade prior. If family doctors, as noted in the recommendation on embracing virtual care, do not adopt this mode of care delivery as a regular part of their workday, you can bet the health care corporations trying to disrupt primary care, including pharmacy chains like CVS Health and big tech companies like Amazon, will take it over.

Another part of the post-pandemic new normal in US primary care will be the increasing embrace of "home" health care. Traditionally, we think of home health care as providing services to elderly patients who cannot get out and require various support or medical services on a regular basis. The pandemic will redefine home health care to mean an array of different services, including primary care services, delivered to populations of all ages. This is where companies like Amazon and Google, who already have the technology in people's homes to connect with them, will flourish. It is also where the nascent trend of personalized health care, aided by wearable technology such as fitness watches, finds a clear purpose.

The pandemic has laid the groundwork for patients to think about receiving all sorts of advice, care management, and care provision in their homes. From Alexa helping them triage their child's recent cut to the Apple Watch recording and uploading vitals such as a person's blood pressure or blood sugar so that they can get real-time guidance on whether they should visit a medical office, our understanding of home health care is going to shift rapidly over the next several years. Chronic disease management, urgent care, medical advice, medication management, triage for different medical conditions: this is what home health is moving toward, spurred by a pandemic that has forced many to remain in their homes and avoid visits to a physician's office unless it was absolutely necessary. Big tech has been waiting for a disruptive event that shows people the value of their gadgets for delivering health care conveniently. COVID-19 is that disruptive event. Patients will end up trying things, like they have done with telehealth, that normally they would have preferred not trying or did not think about ever trying. Family doctors must not be left out of this shift to providing more care in the home setting. They must get involved in being the experts controlling how medical information and care is dispensed through the virtual realm.

Finally, there is a bigger-picture implication of the COVID-19 pandemic for family doctors. As more people delay going to a doctor and getting needed care, how many of them will continue to forget what it is that a family doctor might do for them? For a specialty that struggled to gain relevance in the eyes of patients before, a long pandemic has not helped their cause. Some patients will undoubtedly downplay their need for primary care services moving forward, in part because the pandemic has taught them a misguided lesson that they can go without seeing a doctor and have nothing immediately happen to them. Some will perhaps get more cynical toward a health care system that made many mistakes in dealing with COVID-19 and that showed its general unpreparedness in meeting patients' needs. This cynicism, as well as an overall fatigue with thinking about all things health and medical care, may create individuals who simply see prevention and staying healthy in one of two ways: either as (a) personal and solitary endeavors not requiring much if any interaction with a doctor, or as (b) a series of personal sacrifices and activities difficult to engage in and containing high degrees of uncertainty.

In either of the above scenarios, those individuals will withdraw somewhat from active involvement in the health care system. They will see primary care and family doctors as less central to their own health, not as the difference makers the specialty pitches to them. We may get healthier individuals in American society because of the pandemic. At the same time, we may also get unhealthier individuals. Both groups, for different reasons, could turn away from doctors and primary care medicine. One group may see control over their health as entirely within their own purview, choosing to take more on themselves and see doctors less. The other group may see control over their health as an impossible task for them or anyone else to perform and choose to neglect accessing the health system for all but the most acute issues.

Add to this reality the increasing scarcity of family doctors in many parts of the United States, and the fact that it is harder to gain access to them than ever before because of pandemic restrictions, and their disappearance from view grows more pronounced. The use of more convenient urgent care centers and retail health clinics, accessible now in most every town with the possible exception of rural America, provides an in-your-face care option for many that is hard to pass up. As care delivery moves away from family physicians' offices to other outlets, family doctors will continue to lose ground. In short, the pandemic and its fallout do no favors for the specialty of family practice.

I would like to believe family doctors and the specialty of family practice will effectively reassert their moral and intellectual legitimacy over our primary care system. But I am a realist too. It is one thing to put band-aids on a wound that is not healing, to protect it a bit and hope that it will not get worse. It is quite another to understand that the time for band-aids is well past and more drastic steps must be taken to promote the healing process. The specialty of family medicine and its leaders have, for decades, been applying band-aids when they should have been taking more drastic steps. Where smaller interventions might have worked before, now the treatment approach seems to call for riskier, bigger alternatives.

Having studied the health care system for decades, and having worked in it myself, I believe wholeheartedly in the value of primary care for all of us. To that end, I also believe that the ideal of the comprehensive or generalist family doctor is perhaps the noblest and most human embodiment of the concept of healing that we have in medicine. I have worked with, studied, and gotten to know so many family doctors, and pretty much without exception they are compassionate, competent, and dedicated individuals. Personally, I have rooted for their success my entire adult life, ever since I worked in a department of family practice in my early twenties. If I place any hope in the idea that our health care system can become better for patients, it is based in part on my hope that family doctors can make a significant contribution to achieving that goal.

But as a realist, and as a social scientist who has studied all of this for a long time now, objectively I am less optimistic—unless, of course, the specialty of family practice makes several meaningful changes over the next decade and individual family doctors decide to take more risks with their careers. I dread the large health care corporations and the tech companies moving in to take over primary care. Are these companies here to stay? It's hard to know. But the road to conquering primary care will be easier for them with no strong family doctor army in their way forcing negotiation and compromise.

I place zero confidence in the rest of the medical profession coming to the aid of family medicine. Would you? There is too much bad blood between primary care and the other specialties. There are too many turf issues still outstanding and too many interests of the other medical specialties that may be undermined by a strong family doctor contingent. I do not see how insurance companies, or the government, or employers, who still pay most of the health care bill for people, will use their immense power to sway the system in a direction favoring physician-centric primary care. The name of the game now is access, convenience, and cheaper care. That is what government payers like Medicare and employers want from the delivery system. Family doctors might be able to help with those things, but only if there are a lot more of them in circulation and they can live up to what the role asks.

As I write this coda, I think back again to all those patient letters I read that were given to Richard Rutland, *Good Housekeeping*'s 1981 Family Doctor of the Year, upon his retirement. They included so much admiration for a family doctor, so many feelings of trust and goodwill by patients toward a clinician, and so many thank-yous for things he did for them—the time spent, the attention paid, the respect, the listening, and the empathy. Going the extra mile and helping people make the best medical decisions and letting them know there was someone there who could serve as a guide in their health care journey, Dr. Rutland was the manifestation of the comprehensive family doctor in everyday life. The generalist physician we all need. He was one of many family doctors during that time and since who have embraced this difficult yet rewarding role, making many personal and family sacrifices in the process. Those letters are as sincere a thing as I have seen in my time working in and studying the health care system. The work Rutland put in to leave the legacy he did is undeniable.

This is the main question I ask myself as I think on all this—is our health care system and the specialty of family practice even capable of producing more than just a few Richard Rutlands here and there anymore? I think I know what my answer is to that question, but I try to believe I do not know. In that sense, I continue to hope that all of us can keep the vision of Nick Pisacano and Gayle Stephens in our minds, even if we do not see it in front of us right now. There are many powers in health care that want us to forget, but forgetting that vision will have consequences for us. It moves us one step closer to a colder, more impersonal, and less humane brand of health care. It moves health care one step closer to fast food and online shopping. So much in our lives has lost the human feel to it, and with that the loss of precious qualities we need to thrive as a society, like trust and empathy, that I feel that if we lose health care, there really is nothing left that cannot be swallowed whole by corporate notions of efficiency and technological superiority.

We cannot lose primary care or health care to that end.

A Note on the Research

The research for this book comes from archival research and seventy in-depth interviews with fifty-five different family physicians. These family physicians are from a range of different jobs, settings, organizations, and geographic locales. The archival research is historical in nature, and I was helped tremendously by my access to documents stored at the Center for the History of Family Medicine (CHFM), which is operated by the American Academy of Family Physicians (AAFP) Foundation. The CHFM provided me access to most of their stored documents at the national headquarters of the AAFP in Leawood, Kansas. I visited their facility two times during 2019 and 2020 to examine documents. I also benefited from receiving the Sandra Panther Fellowship from the AAFP Foundation, which provided me with the support to travel there.

What led me to want to draw upon these two distinct sources of data for this project? For one, I never do any research project anymore without relying on qualitative data for at least some of it. I believe, and I have found, that talking to people tells you a lot about reality. The way it is rather than the way people want it to be. Talking with physicians tells you a lot about their everyday world. One that we do not get to see often. Doctors are elite professionals. Things like their fears, anxieties, frustrations, joys, and hopes are normally hidden from view because, as elites, they cannot easily open up about these things without looking human, and many of us want to see our doctors as more than human. Doctors are also a breed of professional that tend to be less self-reflective on the surface. Many do not complain overtly about their personal trials and tribulations. Conducting interviews with physicians where some time is taken to get them to feel comfortable opening up creates the potential for gaining insights into what makes each of them tick. Doctors are also smart individuals. Once they open up a bit, they are some of the most cerebral people you can hope to meet. That helps me better understand what it is I am hearing from them.

Using historical data on the family medicine specialty was somewhat new for me as a researcher. I am not a historian by training; I am an organizational and medical sociologist, more of a social anthropologist. But I have always wanted to do a larger research project that takes advantage of historical data. This project was perfect for realizing that goal. Add to this the good fortune to have a medical specialty in which I was interested possess a repository of historical information about themselves spanning back to the mid-twentieth century, and it made it a no-brainer for me to include this archival research in the project.

The Family Physician Interview Sample

The fifty-five family doctors interviewed for this book were selected purposefully based on my desire to achieve a balance of age, gender, career stage, type of work or employment setting, and geographic location. This was to ensure that any patterns emerging from the interviews might achieve some level of generality across family doctors as a group. The doctors worked primarily in the New York and New England areas of the United States. But most were born and raised somewhere else. Forty-one of the fifty-five doctors were post-residency. Six were medical students who either had already decided to choose family practice or were considering it. Twenty-four of the fifty-five doctors were women. Twelve of the fifty-five were from non-white racial/ethnic backgrounds. Three interviewees were first-year family medicine residents. Five interviewees were either second- or third-year residents. The rest were fully licensed family doctors at various stages of their careers. I interviewed ones starting out in their careers; ones in the middle stages of their careers; and ones in the twilight of their careers. I captured physician ages in the interview sample ranging from 22 to 78 years of age. It was a diverse group of individuals.

Seven of the fifty-five family doctors I had interviewed for prior research projects. However, the vast majority were new interviewees who I had not previously met. I recruited these individuals with the gracious help of the New York State Academy of Family Physicians (NYAFP). The NYAFP allowed me to place a small advertisement in one of their newsletters soliciting recruits for this study. Better yet, they let me attend one of their biannual conferences where I had a table near the conference registration table and could approach family doctors on the spot to try and secure an interview day and time with them. At one conference, I was able to interview eleven family doctors over a span of two days. In addition, I left that conference with the contact information for another ten potential interviewees. I went to a second NYAFP conference six months later and signed up another fifteen interviewees which I was able to interview by phone over the next several months after that conference. The remaining interviewees came through recommendations from the family doctors I interviewed previously.

I made sure not to overload the sample with one type of family doctor or another. The first thing people usually say about qualitative research, particularly when they want to question the results of a given research study, is that the sample is somehow biased or not representative enough. Either I spoke with too many of this type of doctor, or not enough of that type of doctor. But anyone who does a lot of good qualitative research involving interviews knows that if you choose your interviewees wisely—that is, on whether they possess key characteristics which you believe are relevant to understanding the research questions at hand, and whether they are willing to open up and give you rich detail on the phenomena of interest—an interview sample of twenty-five people often yields as good an interpretation as an interview sample of one hundred people. Usually in my research studies, the story I hear rarely changes significantly after the first twenty-five to fifty interviews. Often, that story is one that resonates across the entire group of people I could have interviewed.

In particular, I made sure, though most of the doctors worked in the New York State/New England region, that they worked in a variety of geographic locations: urban, suburban, and rural. In this way, the sample reflected every type of community in which family doctors work. While a rural part of New York State may not be wholly identical to a rural part of North Dakota, they are similar enough that the types of clinical work should be comparable in most instances. As far as how individual family doctors think about themselves or their work, many family doctors are never from the places where they ultimately end up working; they are born and raised somewhere else. Thus, a particular geographic location does not necessarily denote that a given group of doctors will all think the same and share the same values. I recorded and transcribed physician interviews, then used systematic analytic techniques and a special coding software to identify the key themes emanating from the interview data.

The Archival Historical Data

The archival data I reviewed at the Center for the History of Family Medicine included but was not limited to the following: (a) patient letters to Richard Rutland upon his retirement from family medicine practice; (b) select annual reports of the American Academy of General Practice (AAGP) and the American Academy of Family Physicians from 1948 to 1980; (c) committee reports, summaries, personal reflections, and meeting minutes from major AAGP and AAFP initiatives such as the Keystone 1, 2, and 3 conferences and the Future of Family Medicine project; (d) the writings and publications of intellectual leaders such as Nicholas Pisacano and Gayle Stephens; (e) numerous articles about general practice and family medicine published in peer-reviewed journals from 1950 to 2020; (f) major reports such as the Millis Report that helped to lay the groundwork for creating the specialty of family medicine; (g) various published critiques of both the fields of general and family practice written by a variety of authors from the 1950s to the 2010s; (h) facts and trends published about family/general practice, family/general practice work, and family/general doctors over a seventy-year time span; and (i) published histories of organizations like the American Board of Family Medicine.

It should be noted that the CHFM houses a lot of documents, and there is a detailed catalog where you can see the names of these documents. But until you begin reading and examining any particular piece of material, you are not sure what you are going to find. Reviewing some of the donated personal documents for several well-known family doctors and general practitioners was very rewarding. That is how I found out about Richard Rutland, and, in reading about his life and work, found a model for the comprehensive physician ideal the specialty of family practice was hoping to create. But with so much material available, I had to either skim or read more carefully many different documents that looked interesting or potentially relevant. It turns out that a lot of the material was not relevant for this project. But a good amount of it was. Fortunately, I was able to photocopy a lot of the material and read it after my trips. This gave me time to think about how different things I was reading might fit together, and how it might help to inform the interview data I was analyzing at the same time. It slowed my thinking down enough to help me craft a deeper analysis about the specialty— where it was headed, how its doctors were evolving, and what that meant for primary care in America.

Crafting the Book

In the end, the story in this book came about through an iterative process of examining and reexamining the relevant data, using the systematic methods a good qualitative researcher has at their disposal. These include the use of coding software to help identify patterns and themes, content analysis of various chunks of text embedded in documents and interview transcripts, theoretical sampling that allowed me to make decisions on which phenomena should be investigated further with additional data, and triangulating findings from different data sources to help determine the right interpretations to make. I have done a lot of qualitative research in my career, and I feel confident the analytic approach I took for this project was sound.

The writing of this book's manuscript occurred simultaneously with the data collection and analysis. I created initial outlines of various chapters, aligned with the preliminary data analysis that was emerging from the archival and interview data. I cultivated these outlines into more detailed ones, changing the foci and order of chapters in line with how the data analysis was evolving. I also collected additional data over time that called for modifications to several of the chapters. The drafting of the book manuscript went through approximately three very detailed iterations before it was sent to my editor for review. Overall, the entire process, from the beginning of data collection to the completed book manuscript, took almost two years.

What do I think of the interpretation I derived from all these data and the ultimate story it tells? I think the story is sound. It resonates as believable, which is the hallmark of good qualitative research. The interview data triangulate in a close-knit way with what the archival data speak to historically. In other words, it all seems to fit. Some family doctors, or the specialty itself, may recoil at aspects of the findings presented here. They may disagree wholeheartedly with my interpretation. They may think that a lot is left out that would change how this story gets told. Of course, every research project is limited by not having the universe of relevant knowledge on hand to analyze. I am sure there are nuances and aspects of this story that are important, and which I did not cover in this study. Still, I am not sure they would change the fundamental message of this book. In that sense, I will again say I think the story told here is sound. It may not be the entire story, but it is an accurate one given the data at my disposal.

REFERENCES

Preface

Peterson, Stephen, Robert McNellis, Kathleen Klink, David Meyers, and Andrew Bazemore. 2018. The State of Primary Care in the United States: A Chartbook of Facts and Statistics. https://www.graham-center.org/content/dam/rgc/documents /publications-reports/reports/PrimaryCareChartbook.pdf.

Chapter 1

American Academy of Family Physicians. 2019. Joint Statement: Hospitalists Trained in Family Medicine. https://www.aafp.org/practice-management/administration /hospitalists/joint-statement.html.

Basu, Sanjay, Seth A. Berkowitz, Robert L. Phillips, Asaf Bitton, Bruce E. Landon, and Russell S. Phillips. 2019. Association of Primary Care Physician Supply with Population Mortality in the United States, 2005–2015. *JAMA Internal Medicine* 179, no. 4: 506–514. https://doi.org/10.1001/jamainternmed.2018.7624.

Boodman, Sandra. 2018. Spurred by Convenience, Millennials Often Spurn the "Family Doctor" Model. Kaiser Health. https://khn.org/news/spurred-by -convenience-millennials-often-spurn-the-family-doctor-model/.

City of Fayette. 2019. https://fayetteal.org/.

Doximity. 2019. Physician Compensation Report. https://s3.amazonaws.com/s3 .doximity.com/press/doximity_third_annual_physician_compensation_report _round4.pdf.

Frank, Elena, Zhuo Zhao, Srijan Sen, and Constance Guille. 2019. Gender Disparities in Work and Parental Status Among Early Career Physicians. *JAMA Network Open* 2, no. 8: e198340. https://doi.org/10.1001/jamanetworkopen.2019.8340.

Griggs, Mary Beth. 2019. Amazon Is Now Offering Virtual Health Care to Its Employees. The Verge. https://www.theverge.com/2019/9/24/20882335/amazon -care-telemedicine-employees-healthcare.

Hertzler, Arthur E., and Milburn Stone. 1938. *The Horse and Buggy Doctor*. Lincoln: University of Nebraska Press.

Hoff, Timothy J. 2010. *Practice Under Pressure: Primary Care Physicians and Their Medicine in the Twenty-First Century*. New Brunswick, NJ: Rutgers University Press.

Hoff, Timothy J. 2017. *Next in Line: Lowered Care Expectations in the Age of Retail- and Value-Based Health*. Oxford: Oxford University Press.

Landi, Heather. 2019. CVS Health Exec: Retail Giant Wants to Create a Netflix-like Healthcare Experience. Fierce Healthcare. https://www.fiercehealthcare.com/tech

/cvs-health-s-digital-executive-we-want-to-create-a-healthcare-experience-as-easy
-to-use-and.

Medscape. 2018. 2018 Family Physician Compensation Report. https://www.medscape
.com/slideshow/2018-compensation-family-physician-6009655.

Merritt Hawkins. 2017. Survey of Physician Appointment Wait Times. https://www
.merritthawkins.com/uploadedFiles/MerrittHawkins/Content/Pdf/mha2017wait
timesurveyPDF.pdf.

Millis, John S. 1966. The Millis Commission Report. Chicago: American Medical
Association.

National Resident Matching Program. 2019. Main Residency Match Data and Reports.
http://www.nrmp.org/main-residency-match-data/.

Physicians Foundation. 2018. 2018 Survey of America's Physicians. https://physicians
foundation.org/wp-content/uploads/2018/09/physicians-survey-results-final-2018
.pdf.

RAND. 2016. The Evolving Role of Retail Clinics. Santa Monica, CA: RAND
Corporation. https://www.rand.org/pubs/research_briefs/RB9491-2.html.

Stephens, G. Gayle. 1989. Family Medicine as Counterculture. *Family Medicine* 21,
no. 2: 103–109.

Chapter 2

American Medical Association. 2020a. RBRVS Overview. https://www.ama-assn.org
/about/rvs-update-committee-ruc/rbrvs-overview.

American Medical Association. 2020b. RVS Update Committee (RUC). https://www
.ama-assn.org/about/rvs-update-committee-ruc.

Babylon Health. 2019. AI. https://www.babylonhealth.com/ai.

Basu, Sanjay, Russell S. Phillips, Zirui Song, Bruce E. Landon, and Asaf Bitton. 2016.
Effects of New Funding Models for Patient-Centered Medical Homes on Primary
Care Practice Finances and Services: Results of a Microsimulation Model. *Annals
of Family Medicine* 14, no. 5: 404–414.

Bazemore, Andrew W., Laura A. Makaroff, James C. Puffer, Parwen Parhat, Robert L.
Phillips, Imam M. Xierali, and Jason Rinaldo. 2012. Declining Numbers of Family
Physicians Are Caring for Children. *Journal of the American Board of Family
Medicine* 25, no. 2: 139–140.

Berenson, Robert A., and Eugene C. Rich. 2010. US Approaches to Physician
Payment: The Deconstruction of Primary Care. *Journal of General Internal
Medicine* 25, no. 6: 613–618. https://doi.org/10.1007/s11606-010-1295-z.

Berwick, Donald M. 1996. Payment by Capitation and the Quality of Care. *New
England Journal of Medicine* 335: 1227–1231.

Bodenheimer, Thomas, Robert A. Berenson, and Paul Rudolf. 2007. The Primary
Care–Specialty Income Gap: Why It Matters. *Annals of Internal Medicine* 146,
no. 4: 301–306.

Casalino, Lawrence P., David Gans, Rachel Weber, Meagan Cea, Amber Tuchovsky,
Tara F. Bishop, Yesenia Miranda, et al. 2016. US Physician Practices Spend More
Than $15.4 Billion Annually to Report Quality Measures. *Health Affairs* 35,
no. 3: 401–406.

Coutinho, Anastasia J., Anneli Cochrane, Keith Stelter, Robert L. Phillips, and Lars E.
Peterson. 2015. Comparison of Intended Scope of Practice for Family Medicine

Residents with Reported Scope of Practice Among Practicing Family Physicians. *JAMA* 314, no. 22: 2364. https://doi.org/10.1001/jama.2015.13734.

Dorsey, E. Ray, David Jarjoura, and Gregory W. Rutecki. 2003. Influence of Controllable Lifestyle on Recent Trends in Specialty Choice by US Medical Students. *JAMA* 290, no. 9: 1173–1178.

Farr, Christina. 2018. Amazon and Apple Are Getting into Medical Clinics—Here's Why. CNBC online. https://www.cnbc.com/2018/09/08/amazon-and-apple-are-getting-into-medical-clinics-heres-why.html.

Friedman, Emily. 1996. Capitation, Integration, and Managed Care: Lessons from Early Experiments. *JAMA* 275, no. 12: 957–962.

Hoff, Timothy J. 2010. *Primary Care Physicians and Their Medicine in the Twenty-first Century*. New Brunswick, NJ: Rutgers University Press.

Hoff, Timothy J. 2011. Deskilling and Adaptation among Primary Care Physicians Using Two Work Innovations. *Health Care Management Review* 36, no. 4: 338–348. https://doi.org/10.1097/HMR.0b013e31821826a1.

Hoff, Timothy J. 2017. *Next in Line: Lowered Care Expectations in the Age of Retail- and Value-Based Health*. Oxford: Oxford University Press.

Huckman, Robert. 2019. Can Big-Box Retailers Provide Local Health Care? *Harvard Business Review*. https://hbr.org/2019/10/can-big-box-retailers-provide-local-health-care.

Japsen, Bruce. 2019. CVS Profits Rise as Health Hubs Open. Forbes. https://www.forbes.com/sites/brucejapsen/2019/11/06/cvs-profits-rise-as-health-hubs-open-and-aetna-deal-takes-hold/#6fe18162574e.

Kane, Carole K. 2019. Updated Data on Physician Practice Arrangements: For the First Time, Fewer Physicians Are Owners Than Employees. AMA Economic and Health Policy Research. https://www.ama-assn.org/sites/ama-assn.org/files/corp/media-browser/public/health-policy/PRP-2016-physician-benchmark-survey.pdf.

Kerr, Eve A., Ron D. Hays, Allison Mitchinson, Martin Lee, and Albert L. Siu. 1999. The Influence of Gatekeeping and Utilization Review on Patient Satisfaction. *Journal of General Internal Medicine* 14, no. 5: 287–296.

Kruse, Clemens Scott, Caitlin Kristof, Beau Jones, Erica Mitchell, and Angelica Martinez. Barriers to Electronic Health Record Adoption: A Systematic Literature Review. *Journal of Medical Systems* 40, no. 12. https://doi.org/10.1007/s10916-016-0628-9.

Langenbrunner, John C., Deborah K. Williams, and Sherry A. Terrell. 1988. Physician Incomes and Work Patterns across Specialties: 1975 and 1983–84. *Health Care Financing Review* 10, no. 2: 17–24. https://www.ncbi.nlm.nih.gov/pmc/articles/PMC4192917/.

LaPointe, Jacqueline. 2019. Hospital Acquisitions of Physician Practices Rose 128 Percent Since 2012. RevCycle Intelligence. https://revcycleintelligence.com/news/hospital-acquisitions-of-physician-practices-rose-128-since-2012.

Mazzolini, Chris. 2019. Employed Physicians Outnumber Independent Physicians for the First Time Ever. Medical Economics. https://www.medicaleconomics.com/news/employed-physicians-outnumber-independent-physicians-first-time-ever.

Merritt Hawkins. 2017. Survey of Physician Appointment Wait Times. https://www.merritthawkins.com/uploadedFiles/MerrittHawkins/Content/Pdf/mha2017wait timesurveyPDF.pdf.

National Committee for Quality Assurance. 2019. Patient-Centered Recognition Programs. https://www.ncqa.org/education-training/webinars-and-seminars/patient-centered-medical-home-pcmh/.

Neumann, Kane, Andrew Bazemore, and Ann Greiner. Investing in Primary Care: A State-Level Analysis. PCPCC Annual Evidence Report. Patient-Centered Primary Care Collaborative. Robert Graham Center. https://www.pcpcc.org/sites/default/files/resources/pcmh_evidence_es_2019.pdf.

Ortiz-Ospina, Esteban, and Max Roser. 2019. Financing Healthcare. Our World in Data. https://ourworldindata.org/financing-healthcare.

Osborn, Robin, Donald Moulds, Eric C. Schneider, Michelle M. Doty, David Squires, and Dana O. Sarnak. 2015. Primary Care Physicians in Ten Countries Report Challenges Caring for Patients with Complex Health Needs. *Health Affairs* 34, no. 12: 2104–2112. https://doi.org/10.1377/hlthaff.2015.1018.

Physicians Foundation. 2018 Survey of America's Physicians. https://physiciansfoundation.org/wp-content/uploads/2018/09/physicians-survey-results-final-2018.pdf.

Rama, A. 2018. Policy Research Perspectives, Payment and Delivery in 2018. American Medical Association. https://www.ama-assn.org/system/files/2019-09/prp-care-delivery-payment-models-2018.pdf.

RAND. 2016. The Evolving Role of Retail Clinics. RAND Corporation. https://www.rand.org/pubs/research_briefs/RB9491-2.html.

Rege, Alyssa. 2017. AMA: 92% of Millennial Physicians Cite Work-Life Balance as a Priority. Becker's Hospital Review. https://www.beckershospitalreview.com/hospital-physician-relationships/ama-92-of-millennial-physicians-cite-work-life-balance-as-a-priority.html.

Robertson, Ruth, Sarah Gregory, and Joni Jabbal. 2014. The Social Care and Health System of Nine Countries. Commission on the Future of Health and Social Care in England. https://pdfs.semanticscholar.org/90f4/f806496564a45667d7bbe73bfb01872cf365.pdf.

Rosenthal, Elisabeth. 2018. An American Sickness: How Health Care Became Big Business and How You Can Take It Back. *Missouri Medicine* 115, no. 2: 128.

Shanafelt, Tait D., Omar Hasan, Lotte N. Dyrbye, Christine Sinsky, Daniel Satele, Jeff Sloan, and Colin P. West. 2015. Changes in Burnout and Satisfaction with Work-Life Balance in Physicians and the General US Working Population between 2011 and 2014. *Mayo Clinic Proceedings* 90, no. 12: 1600–1613. https://doi.org/10.1016/j.mayocp.2015.08.023.

Starr, Paul. 1982. *The Social Transformation of American Medicine*. New York: Basic Books.

Tong, Sebastian T. C., Laura A. Makaroff, Imam M. Xierali, Parwen Parhat, James C. Puffer, Warren P. Newton, and Andrew W. Bazemore. 2012. Proportion of Family Physicians Providing Maternity Care Continues to Decline. *Journal of the American Board of Family Medicine* 25, no. 3: 270–271.

Tong, Sebastian T., Laura A. Makaroff, Imam M. Xierali, James C. Puffer, Warren P. Newton, and Andrew W. Bazemore. 2013. Family Physicians in the Maternity Care Workforce: Factors Influencing Declining Trends. *Maternal and Child Health Journal* 17, no. 9: 1576–1581. https://link.springer.com/article/10.1007/s10995-012-1159-8.

Tosto, Amanda. 2019. Who Will Be the Winner in This Digital Health Arms Race? The Hill. https://thehill.com/opinion/healthcare/468531-who-will-be-the-winner-in-this-digital-health-arms-race.

Wachter, Robert M., and Lee Goldman. 2016. Zero to 50,000—the 20th Anniversary of the Hospitalist. *New England Journal of Medicine* 375, no. 11: 1009–1011. https://doi.org/10.1056/nejmp1607958.

Weidner, Amanda K. H., and Frederick M. Chen. Changes in Preparation and Practice Patterns among New Family Physicians. *Annals of Family Medicine* 17, no. 1: 46–48. https://doi.org/10.1370/afm.2337.

Yarnall, Kimberly S. H., Kathryn I. Pollak, Truls Østbye, Katrina M. Krause, and J. Lloyd Michener. 2003. Primary Care: Is There Enough Time for Prevention? *American Journal of Public Health* 93, no. 4: 635–664.

Chapter 3

De Vos, Ans, and Beatrice I. J. M. Van der Heijden. 2015. *Handbook of Research on Sustainable Careers*. Cheltenham, UK: Edward Elgar Publishing.

De Vos, Ans, Beatrice I. J. M. Van der Heijden, and Jos Akkermans. 2018. Sustainable Careers: Towards a Conceptual Model. *Journal of Vocational Behavior*. https://www.sciencedirect.com/science/article/pii/S0001879118300769?via%3Dihub.

Lawrence, Barbara S., Douglas T. Hall, and Michael B. Arthur. 2015. Sustainable Careers Then and Now. In *Handbook of Research on Sustainable Careers*, edited by Beatrice I. J. M. Van der Heijden, 432–450. Cheltenham, UK: Edward Elgar Publishing.

Chapter 4

American Academy of Family Physicians. n.d. Rep. Timeline of Significant AAFP Events.

American Academy of Family Physicians. 1980. Rep. Creation of a Specialty.

American Academy of General Practice. 1948a. Rep. Committee on Education. Annual Report.

American Academy of General Practice. 1948b. Rep. Distribution and Type of Practice of Members of the American Academy of General Practice.

American Academy of General Practice. 1957. Data on Academy Members. Internal Memo.

American Academy of General Practice. 1958. Rep. Study of Practice Patterns of Members of the American Academy of General Practice.

American Academy of General Practice. 1966. Rep. The Core Content of Family Medicine. *General Practice*: 225–245.

Canadian Family Physician. 1989. AMFP Head: No FP-IM Merger "as Long as I Can Breathe."

Hamburg, J. 1990. In Memoriam, Nicholas Pisacano. Center for the History of Family Medicine archives. University of Kentucky Medical Center. Lexington, KY.

Journal of the American Medical Association. 1990. Obituaries. *JAMA* 264, no. 4: 445.

Millis, John S. 1966. The Millis Commission Report. Chicago: American Medical Association.

Pisacano, Nicholas J. 1964. General Practice: A Eulogy. *General Practice* 29: 173–181.

Pisacano, Nicholas J. 1966. Family Practice as a Specialty. Center for the History of Family Medicine archives. University of Kentucky Medical Center. Lexington, KY.

Pisacano, Nicholas J. 1970. Trends in Graduate Education. Talk Delivered to the Association for Hospital Medical Education at the American Medical Association Annual Congress.

Rodnick, J. E. 1987. A Brief History of STFM: Reflections on Our First Decade, 1967–1977. *Family Medicine* 19, no. 5: 386–387.

Starr, Paul. 1982. *The Social Transformation of American Medicine*. New York: Basic Books.

Stephens, G. Gayle. 2010. Remembering 40 Years, Plus or Minus. *Journal of the American Board of Family Medicine* 23, supplement: S5–S10. https://doi.org/10.3122 /jabfm.2010.s1.090293.

Young, Paul R. 1995. A Brief History of the American Board of Family Practice. *Journal of the American Board of Family Medicine* 9, no. 2: 109–113.

Chapter 5

American Academy of Family Physicians. 1971. Annual Report.

American Academy of Family Physicians. 1976. Annual Report.

American Academy of Family Physicians. 1999. Keystone III Conference Roundtable.

American Academy of General Practice. 1966. Rep. The Core Content of Family Medicine. *General Practice*: 225–245.

American Medical Association. 1968. Rep. Essentials for Residency Training in Family Practice. Department of Graduate Medical Education.

Family Health Foundation of America. 1969. *The Role of the Family Physician in America's Developing Medical Care Program*. St. Louis: W. H. Green.

Millis, John S. 1966. The Millis Commission Report. Chicago: American Medical Association.

Phillips, Robert L., Stacy Brungardt, Sarah E. Lesko, Nathan Kittle, Jason E. Marker, Michael L. Tuggy, Michael L. LeFevre, et al. 2014. The Future Role of the Family Physician in the United States: A Rigorous Exercise in Definition. *Annals of Family Medicine* 12, no. 3: 250–255.

Pisacano, Nicholas J. 1964. General Practice: A Eulogy. *General Practice* 29: 173–181.

Pisacano, Nicholas J. 1966. Family Practice as a Specialty. Center for the History of Family Medicine archives. University of Kentucky Medical Center. Lexington, KY.

Pisacano, Nicholas J. 1970. Generally Speaking. *JAMA* 213, no. 3: 432–433.

Chapter 6

Gaynor, Martin. 2018. Examining the Impact of Health Care Consolidation. Statement before the Committee on Energy and Commerce, Oversight and Investigations Subcommittee, US House of Representatives. February 14, 2018.

Hoff, Timothy J. 2017. *Next in Line: Lowered Care Expectations in the Age of Retail- and Value-Based Health*. Oxford: Oxford University Press.

Starr, Paul. 1982. *The Social Transformation of American Medicine*. New York: Basic Books.

Chapter 8

American Academy of Family Physicians. 1971. Annual Report.

American Academy of Family Physicians. 1974. Annual Report.

American Academy of Family Physicians. 1976. Annual Report.

American Academy of Family Physicians. 2000a. Practice Profile I Survey.

American Academy of Family Physicians. 2000b. Practice Profile II Survey.

American Academy of Family Physicians. 2020a. 2020 Match Results for Family Medicine. https://www.aafp.org/medical-school-residency/program-directors/nrmp.html.

American Academy of Family Physicians. 2020b. Career Options in Family Medicine. https://www.aafp.org/medical-school-residency/choosing-fm/practice.html.

American Academy of Family Physicians. 2020c. Family Medicine: Comprehensive Care for the Whole Person. https://www.aafp.org/medical-school-residency/choosing-fm/model.html.

American Medical Association. 1988. The Future of Family Practice: Implications of the Changing Environment of Medicine. Council on Long Range Planning and Development. *JAMA* 260, no. 9: 1272–1279.

Association of American Medical Colleges. 2020. The Complexities of Physician Supply and Demand: Projections from 2018 to 2033. https://www.aamc.org/system/files/2020-06/stratcomm-aamc-physician-workforce-projections-june-2020.pdf.

Brown, Steven R., and Gretchen Irwin. 2018. Measuring and Improving Continuity in Residency Primary Care Practice. *Annals of Family Medicine* 16, no. 3: 273–274. https://doi.org/10.1370/afm.2250.

Center for the History of Family Medicine. 2019. A Pocket History of Family Medicine in the United States. Leawood, KS: American Academy of Family Physicians Foundation.

Coutinho, Anastasia J., Anneli Cochrane, Keith Stelter, Robert L. Phillips, and Lars E. Peterson. 2015. Comparison of Intended Scope of Practice for Family Medicine Residents with Reported Scope of Practice among Practicing Family Physicians. *JAMA* 314, no. 22: 2364–2372. https://doi.org/10.1001/jama.2015.13734.

Future of Family Medicine. 2004. The Future of Family Medicine: A Collaborative Project of the Family Medicine Community. *Annals of Family Medicine* 2, supplement 1: S3–S32. https://doi.org/10.1370/afm.130.

Hoff, Timothy J. 2010. *Primary Care Physicians and Their Medicine in the Twenty-first Century*. New Brunswick, NJ: Rutgers University Press.

Hurt, Jeannette. 2017. Medical Residents Angered at Extended Work Hours. Medical Economics. https://www.medicaleconomics.com/view/medical-residents-angered-extended-work-hours.

Pisacano, Nicholas J. 1990. Twenty Years: More Questions than Answers *Non Amo Te. Journal of the American Board of Family Medicine* 3, no. 1: 63–65. https://www.jabfm.org/content/3/1/63.2.

Ricketts, Thomas C., Gordon H. DeFriese, and Glenn Wilson. 1986. Trends in the Growth of Family Practice Residency Training Programs. *Health Affairs* 5, no. 4: 84–96. https://doi.org/10.1377/hlthaff.5.4.84.

Stephens, G. Gayle. 1975. The Intellectual Basis of Family Practice. *Family Medicine* 2, no. 6: 423–428. https://www.mdedge.com/familymedicine/article/182649/intellectual-basis-family-practice.

Stephens, G. Gayle. 1979. Family Medicine as Counterculture. *Family Medicine* 21, no. 2: 103–109.

Stephens, G. Gayle. 1981. Family Practice: The Renaissance Is Over. *Journal of the Royal College of General Practitioners* 31, no. 229: 460–466.

Stephens, G. Gayle. 1982. The Case for Family Practice as the Best Model of Primary Care for the U.S. In *The Intellectual Basis of Family Practice*. Tuscon, AZ: Winter Publishing Company.

Stephens, G. Gayle. 2001. Family Practice and Social and Political Change. *Family Medicine* 33, no. 4: 248–251. https://fammedarchives.blob.core.windows.net /imagesandpdfs/pdfs/FamilyMedicineVol33Issue4Stephens248.pdf.

Stephens, G. Gayle. 2010. Remembering 40 Years, Plus or Minus. *Journal of the American Board of Family Medicine* 23, supplement: S5–S10. https://doi.org/10 .3122/jabfm.2010.s1.090293.

Weidner, Amanda K. H., and Frederick Chen. 2019. Changes in Preparation and Practice Patterns among New Family Physicians. *Annals of Family Medicine* 17, no. 1: 46–48. https://doi.org/10.1370/afm.2337.

Willard, William R. 1978. The Challenge of Family Practice Reconsidered. *JAMA* 240, no. 5: 454–458. https://jamanetwork.com/journals/jama/fullarticle /360708.

Chapter 9

Abrams, Ken, and Natasha Elsner. 2018. What Can Health Systems Do to Encourage Physicians to Embrace Virtual Care? *Deloitte Insights*. https://www2.deloitte.com/us /en/insights/industry/health-care/virtual-health-care-health-consumer-and-physician -surveys.html?id=us%3A2el%3A3pr%3A4di4407%3A5awa%3A6di%3AMMDDY Y%3A.

American Academy of Family Physicians. 2020a. Family Physicians Delivering Emergency Medical Care—Critical Challenges and Opportunities. https://www .aafp.org/about/policies/all/family-physicians-emergency-care.html.

American Academy of Family Physicians. 2020b. Nurse Practitioners. https://www .aafp.org/about/policies/all/nurse-practitioners.html.

American Association of Nurse Practitioners. 2020. State Practice Environment. https://www.aanp.org/advocacy/state/state-practice-environment.

American Board of Family Medicine. 2020. Designation of Focused Practice in Hospital Medicine. https://www.theabfm.org/added-qualifications/designation -focused-practice-hospital-medicine.

Amwell. 2019. Telehealth Index: 2019 Physician Survey. https://business.amwell.com /resources/telehealth-index-2019-physician-survey/.

Business Wire. 2015. Family Physicians Say They Would Use Telehealth If Appropri- ately Paid. *Business Wire*. November 16. https://www.businesswire.com/news/home /20151116005977/en/Family-Physicians-Telehealth-Appropriately-Paid.

Centers for Medicare and Medicaid Services. 2020. Trump Administration Makes Sweeping Regulatory Changes to Help U.S. Healthcare System Address COVID-19 Patient Surge. CMS.gov. https://www.cms.gov/newsroom/press-releases/trump -administration-makes-sweeping-regulatory-changes-help-us-healthcare-system -address-covid-19.

Chen, James. 2019. Scarcity Principle. *Investopedia*. https://www.investopedia.com /terms/s/scarcity-principle.asp.

Conradt, Stacy. 2017. 15 Companies that Changed Their Name. Mental Floss. https://www.mentalfloss.com/article/503464/15-companies-changed-their-names.

Dyrbye, Liselotte N., Matthew R. Thomas, and Tait D. Shanafelt. 2006. Systematic Review of Depression, Anxiety, and Other Indicators of Psychological Distress among U.S. and Canadian Medical Students. *Academic Medicine* 81, no. 4: 354–373.

Future of Family Medicine Project Leadership Committee. 2004. The Future of Family Medicine: A Collaborative Project of the Family Medicine Community. *Annals of Family Medicine* 2, supplement 1: S3–S32. https://doi.org/10.1370/afm.130.

Hoff, Timothy J. 2000. Physician Unionization in the United States: Fad or Phenomenon? *Journal of Health and Human Services Administration* 23, no. 1: 5–23. http://www.jstor.org/stable/25780933.

Hoff, Timothy J. 2010. *Practice under Pressure: Primary Care Physicians and Their Medicine in the Twenty-First Century*. New Brunswick, NJ: Rutgers University Press.

Hoff, Timothy J. 2017. *Next in Line: Lowered Care Expectations in the Age of Retail- and Value-Based Health*. Oxford: Oxford University Press.

Hoff, Timothy J. 2018. Medical Training Programs Need to Care about Physician Burnout. Should the Rest of Us? *STAT*. https://www.statnews.com/2018/06/21/medical-training-physician-burnout/.

Hoff, Timothy J. 2020. The Challenges of Consumerism for Primary Care Physicians. *American Journal of Managed Care* 26, no. 1: E1–E3. https://www.ajmc.com/journals/issue/2020/2020-vol26-n1/the-challenges-of-consumerism-for-primary-care-physicians?p=1.

Jonas, Michael. 2018. State Sees Huge Growth of Urgent Care Centers and Retail Clinics. Commonwealth. https://commonwealthmagazine.org/health-care/state-sees-huge-growth-of-urgent-care-centers-and-retail-clinics/.

Joseph, Richard, and Sohan Japa. 2019. We Were Inspired to Become Primary Care Physicians. Now We're Reconsidering a Field in Crisis. *STAT*. https://www.statnews.com/2019/06/20/primary-care-field-crisis/.

Krasniansky, Adriana. 2019. Diving Deeper into Amazon Alexa's HIPAA Compliance. The Hastings Center. https://www.thehastingscenter.org/diving-deeper-into-amazon-alexas-hipaa-compliance/.

Landro, Laura. 2020. How Apps Can Help Manage Chronic Diseases. *Wall Street Journal*. https://partners.wsj.com/ama/charting-change/apps-can-help-manage-chronic-diseases/.

Larry Green Center. 2020. https://www.green-center.org/.

Millis, John S. 1966. The Millis Commission Report. Chicago: American Medical Association.

Politico and Harvard T.H. Chan School of Public Health. 2019. Rep. Americans' Views on Data Privacy and E-Cigarettes. https://cdn1.sph.harvard.edu/wp-content/uploads/sites/94/2019/08/Politico-HSPH-Data-Privacy-E-Cig-Report-081519.pdf.

Ramos, Marco, Tess Lanzarotta, and Iris Chandler. 2020. COVID-19 Is Changing What It Means to Be a Doctor. *Boston Review*. http://bostonreview.net/science-nature/marco-ramos-tess-lanzarotta-iris-chandler-covid-19-changing-what-it-means-be-doctor.

Schoenberg, Shira. 2020. Telehealth Is Burgeoning, But How to Pay for It? Commonwealth. https://commonwealthmagazine.org/health/telehealth-is-burgeoning-but-how-to-pay-for-it/.

Shachar, Carmel, Jaclyn Engel, and Glyn Elwyn. 2020. Implications for Telehealth in a Postpandemic Future. *JAMA* 323, no. 23: 2375–2376. https://doi.org/10.1001/jama.2020.7943.

Union of American Physicians and Dentists. 2020. About UAPD. https://www.uapd.com/about/.

Vahdat, Shaghayegh, Leila Hamzehgardeshi, Somayeh Hessam, and Zeinab Hamzehgardeshi. 2014. Patient Involvement in Health Care Decision Making: A Review. *Iranian Red Crescent Medical Journal* 16, no. 1. https://pubmed.ncbi.nlm.nih.gov/24719703/.

Williams, Andrew. 2020. Apple IOS 13.6 Update Feature Reveals Apple's Play for Patient Medical Records. Forbes. https://www.forbes.com/sites/andrewwilliams/2020/07/17/apple-ios-136-update-feature-reveals-apples-play-for-patient-medical-records/#1ebee1019945.

Witte, Florence M., Terry D. Stratton, and Lois Margaret Nora. 2006. Stories from the Field: Students' Descriptions of Gender Discrimination and Sexual Harassment during Medical School. *Academic Medicine* 81, no. 7: 648–654.

practice, 97–98, 104–9; role of specialty medicine in, 4, 99–100, 109, 112, 194–95; specialist term in, 106–8; as unrealistic, 102–4, 154, 173–74, 194, 197, 203
dissatisfaction. *See* satisfaction/dissatisfaction

electronic health records: burden of, 19, 37, 43, 182; and data sentinel role, 211–15, 222, 225, 241; and dissatisfaction, 37, 43, 44; integrated health records, 210; and retail/"pop-up" model, 42–43
emergency medicine: AAFP on, 224; alliances with, 222, 224–25; community engagement in, 227–28; and general practitioners, 4, 79, 81; and narrowing of scope, 45, 46–47, 48, 181, 189, 190; rise of specialty in, 109; and shift away from family practice, 154, 157, 195, 196, 234
employability, 71
employee model: advocacy and organization in, 218–21; community engagement in, 138–42; and identity, 49; income and compensation, 67, 155, 156, 162; lack of autonomy in, 19–20, 49, 162, 183, 218, 219; owners as employees, 135, 161–66; and realists, 167–68; rise of, ix, 3, 19, 20–22, 48, 202–3; and satisfaction, 49, 140, 143–45; and scope of work, 20, 48–49, 139–40; and shift of infrastructure costs, 37; and true believers, 138–42, 143–45; and work-life balance, 19, 48–49, 144, 145–46, 162, 163
"Essentials for Residency Training in Family Practice," 99–100
evaluation-and-management-services reimbursements, 32–34
exams: certification, 17, 113; medical licensing, 230

family doctors: as data sources, xiii–xiv, xv, 24–25; decline in, 178–80; numbers of, x, 176; public perceptions of, 190, 191, 202, 203, 236, 239,

241–42; as repackaged general practitioners, 76–77, 105–6, 194–95; shortage of, 19, 35, 178, 179, 204–5, 242; as term, 91, 93; trouble in accessing, 204–5. *See also* career choices; career motivations; employee model; satisfaction/dissatisfaction; training of family doctors
"family medicine" term, 16
family practice: accomplishments of, 20; and challenges of social problems, 152–53; as devalued, x, xii, 21, 29–40, 174, 185–86; failure of ideal, 18–23; and feeder system, 21–22, 30, 43–44, 86, 167; growth of, ix, 176–77; importance of, xi, 23–27; *vs.* internal medicine, 184–85, 191, 205; need for action, 201–7; origins of, ix, 16–18, 75–77, 82–94, 97–98, 171–72; prestige of, 101–2, 104, 174, 179, 180, 190, 191, 229; as term, 16, 93–94, 236; at tipping point, xi–xii, 201–2, 239–44. *See also* defining family practice; health care system as hostile to family practice; identity crisis of family practice; marketing of family practice; relationships; training of family doctors
"Family Practice as a Specialty" (Pisacano), 91
fee-for-service reimbursement, 32, 34
flexibility in career choices, 66–72
Future of Family Medicine project, 190–91, 201–2

gatekeeping and managed care, 35–37, 178
general practitioners: autonomy of, 61, 103–4; community engagement of, 1–3, 5–8, 11–15; as competitors, 80–81, 90; decline of, 17, 77–82, 88–94; distancing from family practice, 76, 77, 91, 93–94, 106–9, 197, 235; family doctors as repackaged, 76–77, 105–6, 194–95; and family practice certification, 90; income and compensation, 31, 61–62; media portrayals of, 9–10, 12–13, 102, 177; numbers of, 78, 81–82, 91;

general practitioners (*cont.*)
Pisacano on, 88–89; prestige of, 1–3, 61, 82, 111; and relationships, 9–14, 19, 32–33, 61–62; residency programs for, 79, 80, 110; scope of work, 5, 9–16, 77, 78–79; and specialty certification, 79–80, 84, 89; training, 9, 78–80, 82, 90, 92–93, 110–12; and work-life balance, 7–8
generational differences: in bet-hedging, 70; in flexibility, 68–69; in ownership, 128–30; in relationships, 130–31, 193; and scope of work, 45–46; in work-life balance attitudes, 48, 128–30
guilds, 220–21
gynecology, 47–48, 77, 98, 108, 109

health care system as hostile to family practice: bureaucracy of and lack of control, 19, 30, 174; and buying of private practices, 135, 138–39; family practice as devalued, x, xii, 21, 29–40, 174, 185–86; general, 23, 186, 202–3; and ownership, 119, 120, 121, 123, 125, 132–33, 137; primary health care as undervalued, x, xii, 29–40, 202–3; and realists, 152, 154, 158–59; and resentment, 158–59; and rise of value-based health care, 202. *See also* corporatization of medicine; insurance; reimbursement; scope of work, narrowing
Health Insurance Portability and Accountability Act (HIPAA), 213
holistic medicine, 10–11
home health care, 240–41
home visits, 139, 140
hospitalists: alliances with, 222, 224–25; as alternative career, 3, 4, 22, 195, 234; and narrowing of scope, 47, 167, 189, 190; renaming from inpatient physicians, 237; rise of, 47
hospitals: acquisition/divestment of private practices by, 135; community engagement in, 227–28; and general practitioners, 78, 79; and narrowing of scope, 47, 181; opposition to family practice, 194; as training sites, 22, 114–15, 175, 192–93, 230–31, 232

identity crisis of family practice: and balkanization, x, 72, 168, 195–98, 203; and definition of family practice, 101–2, 104–5, 174–75, 185–87, 189–92, 194–95; and failure of ideal, 18–23; and imitation, 23, 175, 187–95, 197–98; overview of, ix–x, 4, 22–23; and ownership challenges, 128–30. *See also* employee model; marketing of family practice; satisfaction/dissatisfaction; scope of work, narrowing; strategies
imitation: and identity crisis, 23, 175, 187–95, 197–98; in training, 17, 108, 109–15, 175, 192–93, 230–31
income and compensation: and altruists, 60; compared to other specialties, 4, 34–35, 40, 174; and employee model, 67, 155, 156, 162; of general practitioners, 31, 61–62; and ownership, 31, 120, 123, 124–25, 128–30, 164
information. *See* electronic health records; patient information
inpatient physicians. *See* hospitalists
insurance: administrative burden from, 37, 103; and decoupling of costs and value, 31, 32, 34–35, 46; family doctors as expensive labor, 202, 204; and marketing of family practice, 106. *See also* reimbursement
integrated health record, 210
internal medicine, 184–85, 191, 205
internships by general practitioners, 80, 92

Journal of the American Board of Family Practice, 88

Liaison Committee for Specialty Boards, 112

malpractice and narrowing of scope, 45, 47
managed care, 35–37, 178
Marcus Welby, M.D., 9–10, 12–13, 102, 177
marketing of family practice: as bait and switch, 154, 186–87; and counterculture, 17, 18, 188, 189; and definition

of family practice, 97–98, 104–9; and
distancing from general practitioners,
76, 77, 91, 93–94, 105–6, 197, 235; in
early days, 76–77, 85–86, 91, 93–94;
overview of, ix–x; and Pisacano,
107–8, 189; renaming and rebranding
strategy, 235–37; as specialty, ix–x,
17, 93–94, 106–9, 175, 189–92,
197–98; and Stephens, 173–76,
197–98
media portrayals of general practitioners, 9–10, 12–13, 102, 177
medical assistants. See non-physician
providers
medical centers as training sites, 22,
192–93, 230–31, 232. See also hospitals
medical home care, 37–38
medical school: curriculum, 229–30;
funding for family practice, 176; lack
of student interest in family practice,
21, 179–80, 229, 233; lack of student
interest in general practice, 17, 91–92.
See also training of family doctors;
training of general practitioners
Medicare and Medicaid: and increased
interest in primary health care, 17, 20,
76, 82, 87; and record-keeping
burden, 37; and Resource-Based
Relative Value Scale, 33–34
Millis Commission Report: on need for
general practice reform, 83, 84–85,
100; on training, 110, 111, 112, 228

non-physician providers: alliances with,
222–25; burnout in, 225; as disrup-
tion/competition, 21, 40–42, 43; and
downsizing strategy, 235; rise of, 4,
204, 205, 223
nurse practitioners: AAFP on, 223;
alliances with, 222–25; as disruption/
competition, 21, 41; rise of, 4, 205.
See also non-physician providers

obstetrics: in family practice definition,
108; by general practitioners, 77, 79;
and narrowing of scope, 48, 180, 181,
183–84
ownership, private practice: administrative burden of, 37, 120, 125, 127–28,

163; costs of, 37, 123, 124, 125, 127;
decline in, 48; desire to retire or sell,
121, 127, 133, 135–37, 161–66, 219;
economic risk of, 35, 124; income and
compensation, 31, 120, 123, 124–25,
128–30, 164; older owners, 120–23,
128–30, 131–38, 161–66; overview
of, 119–20; and satisfaction, 122–23,
125–26, 128–29, 130–33; and scope
of work, 121, 122; shift to employee
model, 135, 161–66; as untenable, 20,
123, 137, 161–66; younger owners,
123–31, 161–64

partners, patients as, 215–17
patient-centered medical home, 37–38
patient information: data sentinel role,
211–15, 222, 225, 241; ownership of,
212; and patients as partners, 216;
and technology, 210, 211–15
patient management: as devalued, 182,
185–86; dissatisfaction with, 181–82,
183, 184, 186–87, 225; as idealistic,
173–74; and technology, 206; as term,
173–74, 182, 186
pay-for-performance programs, 38
pediatrics: as alternative to family
practice, 72; in family practice
definition, 97; by general practitioners, 77, 79; and narrowing of scope,
45, 181; opposition to family practice
specialty, 80, 85, 86
pedigree as motivation, 63, 65
Pellegrino, Ed, 198
physician assistants: alliances with,
222–25; rise of, 4, 41, 205. See also
non-physician providers
Pisacano, Nicholas: as advocate for
family practice, 83–84, 86–94, 97–98,
171; background and career, 87–88;
criticism of general practitioner
model, 88–89; and defining family
practice, 97–99, 101; and first
residency programs, 88, 112; and
marketing of family practice, 107–8,
189; on stalled growth of family
practice, 178–79; and training, 109,
110, 112, 113–14, 115
"pop-up" facilities, rise of, 4, 41–42

prestige: and career motivations, 62, 63–64, 111, 180, 229; and employee model, 219; of family practice, 101–2, 104, 174, 179, 180, 190, 191, 229; of general practitioners, 1–3, 61, 82, 111; of primary health care, 38, 203; of specialty medicine, 111

preventive care: and capitation, 36; challenges of model, 36; role in family practice, 20, 82–86

primary care physicians: need for and origins of family practice, 82, 83, 85; numbers of, x; shortage of, 40, 41. *See also* family doctors; family practice

primary health care: as challenging, 18–20, 25; conflicting goals of, ix; effect of COVID-19 on, ix, 239–42; and feeder system, 21–22, 30, 43–44, 86, 167; importance of, xi, 23–27; and Medicare/Medicaid, 17, 20, 76, 82, 87; as needing time, 32–33, 44; and origins of family practice, 82, 83, 85–86; prestige of, 38; as undervalued, x, xii, 29–40, 202–3. *See also* corporatization of medicine; family practice; retail medicine; transactional model

privacy, patient, 213, 214

public health, 20

RBRVS (Resource-Based Relative Value Scale), 33–34

realists: desire to sell or retire, 161–66; and feelings of bait and switch, 155–61, 167–68; increase in, 187; overview of, 151–54; shift away from family practice, 152–60, 166–68

recertification, 17, 46

records. *See* administration and paperwork; electronic health records

registered nurses. *See* non-physician providers

reimbursement: Accountable Care Organizations, 38; capitation, 35–37; and disinterest in family practice, 35, 40, 174, 191, 202; for emergency room visits, 46; for evaluation-and-management-services, 32–34; fee-for-service, 32, 34; as lower than other

specialties, 4, 21, 29–40; and managed care, 35–37; and narrowing of scope of work, 34–35, 45, 46–47, 181; need for justification, 19; and patient-centered medical homes, 37–38; for patient management, 182; and patients as partners, 216; pay-for-performance, 38; and private practices, 120, 122, 123; Resource-Based Relative Value Scale, 33–34; for specialists, 29, 32, 33, 34; and technology, 208, 210; for telemedicine, 208, 240; unproven models of, 38–39; "usual and customary" fees, 32

relationships: and accidental doctors, 66, 72; and altruists, 54, 56, 61; as central to family practice, xi; challenges to, in family practice, 19, 20, 181, 182, 202, 204; and employee model, 48–49, 141, 142; and evaluation and management services, 32–33; and general practitioners, 9–14, 19, 32–33, 61–62; generational differences in, 130–31, 193; lack of training on, 22; and patients as partners, 215–17; and private practices, 121, 122, 128–31, 134, 136, 137; in retail and pop-up models, 40, 42; and Rutland, 32–33; strategies for, 225–28; and telemedicine, 209–10

Relative Value Scale Update Committee, 34

Relative Value Unit, 34

resentment: and feelings of bait and switch, 154–61, 167–68, 186–87, 203, 228, 236; of health care system, 158–59; of retail medicine, 145–46

residency programs: AMA guidelines on, 99–100; and cheap labor, 193, 233; in development of family practice, 88, 110, 112–15; downsizing strategy, 233–35; first, 88, 112, 173; for general practitioners, 79, 80, 110; growth of, 176; numbers of unfilled residencies, 21, 177, 233, 235; as unrealistic, 231–32

Resident Match, 177

Resource-Based Relative Value Scale (RBRVS), 33–34

retail medicine: convenience of, 204–5; and COVID-19, 242; and electronic health records, 42–43; and patient acceptance and engagement, 202, 217; "pop-up" facilities, rise of, 4, 41–42; resentment of, 145–46; rise of, x, 21, 40–44, 203; use of non-physician providers, 223

retirement: of owners, 121, 127, 133, 135–37, 162, 164–65; trend to earlier, 22

rotations in training, 230, 231

Ruhe, William, 197

Rutland, Nancy, 15

Rutland, Richard, 150; background, 4, 5; as family doctor, 1–9, 11, 13–16, 32–33, 244; letters to, 1–3, 5–8, 11–16, 28, 32–33, 52, 74, 96, 118, 170, 200, 244

satisfaction/dissatisfaction: and administrative burdens, 37, 43, 44, 202; of altruists, 59; and bait-and-switch feelings, 154–61, 167–68, 186–87, 203, 228, 236; and debt, 62, 156–57, 160; and demands of family practice, 8–9, 19; and employee model, 49, 140, 143–45; of owners, 122–23, 125–26, 128–29, 130–33; with patient management, 181–82, 183, 184, 186–87, 225; of realists, 152–60, 167; of Rutland, 8; of true believers, 122–23, 125–26, 128–29, 130–33, 143–47

scope of work: in development of family practice, 4, 98–100, 102–4, 109, 110, 180, 181; expanding, 225–28; of general practitioners, 5, 9–16, 77, 78–79; generational differences in, 45–46; and ownership, 121, 122; role of specialty medicine in developing, 4, 99–100, 102, 109, 180, 181; as unrealistic, 102–4, 173–74

scope of work, narrowing: and employee model, 20, 48–49, 139–40; generational differences in, 45–46; and reimbursement, 34–35, 45, 46–47, 181; and specialists, 34–35, 44–48, 180–81, 183–85; as undermining of discipline, 174, 180–87, 190, 196; and work-life balance, 44–45, 48

Society of Teachers in Family Medicine, 113, 173, 188–89

specialist medicine: and American Board of Family Practice, 112; as competition for family practice, 100–101, 109; costs of model, 29, 30, 82, 83; and decline in general practitioners, 77, 79–81; general practitioner as specialty, 79–80, 84, 89; imitation of training, 17, 108, 109–15, 175, 192–93, 230–31; income and compensation, 4, 34–35, 40, 174; marketing of, 85; marketing of family practice as, ix–x, 17, 93–94, 106–9, 175, 189–92, 197–98; and narrowing of scope of work, 34–35, 44–48, 180–81, 183–85; public perceptions of, 111, 191–92; reimbursement for, 29, 32, 33, 34; rise of, x, 9–10, 78, 81, 92; role in defining family practice and scope of work, 4, 99–100, 109, 180, 181, 194–95; "specialist" as term, 106–8

Step 1 exam, 230

Stephens, G. Gayle: background and career, 172–73; on counterculture, 18; on "family practice" term, 236; on imitation of specialty medicine, 187–89, 193–94, 197–98; and marketing of family practice, 173–76, 197–98; and origins of family practice, 18, 75–76, 171–72; on patient management, 173–74, 182, 186; on perception of family practice, 203

strategies: alliances with competitors, 221–25; data sentinel role, 211–15, 222, 225, 241; downsizing family practice, 233–35; embracing virtual care, 208–11; expanding scope, 225–28; local organization and advocacy, 218–21, 222, 225; need for, 201–7, 238–39; patients as partners, 215–17; for relationships, 225–28; renaming family practice, 235–37; for training, 227, 228–35

surgery: by general practitioners, 77, 78, 79, 80; and narrowing family practice scope of work, 99–100, 180–81 technology: and COVID-19, 205, 208, 240; as disruption, 21, 40, 42–43, 203, 206; and embracing virtual care, 208–11; and home health care, 240–41; integrated health records, 210; and patient information, 210, 211–15; and patient management, 206; and reimbursement, 208, 210; rise of, x, 4, 203, 243; in transactional model, ix, 42–43; use of in family practice, 205–6, 208–11. *See also* electronic health records

telemedicine: and community engagement, 140; and COVID-19, 205, 208, 240; embracing virtual care, 208–11; reimbursement for, 208, 240

training of family doctors: as appealing, 70; "clinic first" model, 232; in development of family practice, 16, 17, 84, 86–87, 88, 99–100, 109–15; downsizing strategy, 233–35; funding for, 176; as imitating specialist training, 17, 108, 109–15, 175, 230–31; and narrowing of scope, 45–46; procedures in, 114, 180, 192–93, 234; strategies for, 227, 228–35; training sites, 22, 114–15, 175, 192–93, 230–31, 232; as unrealistic, 22, 114–15, 158–59, 160, 175, 180, 192–93, 227, 229–33. *See also* residency programs

training of general practitioners, 9, 78–80, 82, 90, 92–93, 110–12

transactional model: cheap labor in, ix; and employee model, 49; and loss of private practices, 137; *vs.* patient-centered model, ix; rise of, 23–24, 25–26, 40–44, 137; role of family doctors in, 167; technology in, ix, 42–43

true believers: and career crafting, 142–48; challenges for, 132–33; decline in, 187; and employee model, 138–42, 143–45; older, 120–23; overview of, 119–23; younger,

123–31, 138–48. *See also* ownership, private practice

trust: in family doctors, xi, 23–24, 33; in general practitioners, 19, 81; lack of training on, 160; and narrowing of scope, 47; and ownership, 130; and patient information, 212–13, 214; and patients as partners, 216, 217; and telemedicine, 209

Union of American Physicians and Dentists, 220

unions, 220

urgent care centers: and alliances, 222; and balkanization, 195, 196; community engagement in, 227–28; convenience of, 204; and COVID-19, 242; employment in, 3, 22, 67, 68, 152, 153–54, 183, 195, 232, 234; resentment of, 145–46; rise of, 4, 21, 42, 203, 242

"usual and customary" reimbursement, 32

value: decoupling from costs, 31, 32, 34–35, 46; family practice as devalued, x, xii, 21, 29–40, 174, 185–86; and marketing of family practice, 106; and narrowing of scope of work, 34–35; patient management as devalued, 182, 185–86; primary health care as undervalued, x, xii, 29–40, 202–3

value-based health care, 202

wait times, 13, 21, 204, 205

work-life balance: and career choices and changes, 22; and employee model, 19, 48–49, 144, 145–46, 162, 163; of general practitioners, 7–8; generational differences in attitudes, 48, 128–30; and narrowing scope of work, 44–45, 48; and ownership, 125–26, 128–30; and realists, 155–57, 160; and shift away from family practice, 68, 155–57, 160, 203